Foolproof Weight Loss

Other titles in the
Women's Edge Health Enhancement Guide
series:

Women's Edge
HEALTH ENHANCEMENT GUIDE™

Foolproof Weight Loss

*Lose It Fast and Keep
It Off Guaranteed!*

By Diane Kozak, Judith Springer Riddle, and the editors of

PREVENTION
Health Books
for Women

RODALE

NOTICE

This book is intended as a reference volume only, not as a medical manual. The information given here is designed to help you make informed decisions about your health. It is not intended as a substitute for any treatment that may have been prescribed by your doctor. If you suspect that you have a medical problem, we urge you to seek competent medical help.

Printed in the United States of America.
Rodale Inc. makes every effort to use acid-free ∞, recycled paper ♻

Library of Congress Cataloging-in-Publication Data

    Foolproof weight loss : lose it fast and keep it off guaranteed! / by Diane Kozak, Judith Springer Riddle, and the editors of Prevention Health Books for Women.
         p.   cm.—(Women's edge health enhancement guide)
    Includes index.
    ISBN 1–57954–279–4   hardcover
    1. Weight loss.   I. Kozak, Diane.   II. Riddle, Judith Springer.   III. Prevention Health Books for Women.
    IV. Women's edge health enhancement guides.
    RM222.2 .F66   2000
    613.7'045—dc21   00–009752

Distributed to the book trade by St. Martin's Press

2   4   6   8   10   9   7   5   3   1   hardcover

Visit us on the Web at www.rodalebooks.com, or call us toll-free at (800) 848-4735.

RODALE

WE INSPIRE AND ENABLE PEOPLE TO IMPROVE
THEIR LIVES AND THE WORLD AROUND THEM

Foolproof Weight Loss **Staff**

SERIES EDITOR: Debra L. Gordon
WRITERS: Diane Kozak, Judith Springer Riddle
CONTRIBUTING WRITERS: Debra L. Gordon, Deanna Portz, Alison Rice, Cheryl Romano, Marie Elaina Suszynski
ART DIRECTOR: Darlene Schneck
SERIES AND COVER DESIGNER: Lynn N. Gano
PHOTO EDITOR: James A. Gallucci
ILLUSTRATORS: Shawn Banner, Judy Newhouse, Tom Ward
ASSISTANT RESEARCH MANAGERS: Sandra Salera Lloyd, Shea Zukowski
PRIMARY RESEARCH EDITOR: Anita C. Small
LEAD RESEARCHERS: Jennifer S. Kushnier, Elizabeth Shimer
EDITORIAL RESEARCHERS: Molly Donaldson Brown, Karen Jacobs, Mary S. Mesaros, Valerie Rowe, Kirk Swanson, Becky Theodore, Lucille Uhlman
SENIOR COPY EDITOR: Kathy D. Everleth
EDITORIAL PRODUCTION MANAGER: Marilyn Hauptly
LAYOUT DESIGNER: Donna G. Rossi
MANUFACTURING COORDINATORS: Brenda Miller, Jodi Schaffer, Patrick T. Smith

Rodale Healthy Living Books

VICE PRESIDENT AND *PREVENTION* GROUP EDITORIAL DIRECTOR: Anne Alexander
DIRECTOR OF NEW TITLE DEVELOPMENT: Tammerly Booth
DIRECTOR OF SERIES DEVELOPMENT: Gary Krebs
EDITORIAL DIRECTOR: Michael Ward
VICE PRESIDENT AND MARKETING DIRECTOR: Karen Arbegast
PRODUCT MARKETING MANAGER: Guy Maake
BOOK MANUFACTURING DIRECTOR: Helen Clogston
MANUFACTURING MANAGER: Eileen Bauder, Patrick T. Smith
RESEARCH MANAGER: Ann Gossy Yermish
COPY MANAGER: Lisa D. Andruscavage
PRODUCTION MANAGER: Robert V. Anderson Jr.
DIGITAL PROCESSING MANAGERS: Leslie M. Keefe, Thomas P. Aczel
OFFICE MANAGER: Jacqueline Dornblaser
OFFICE STAFF: Susan B. Dorschutz, Julie Kehs Minnix, Tara Schrantz, Catherine E. Strouse

Contents

PART FOUR
The Beat Goes On

Introduction:
The Eternal Quest

Diet. Like any four-letter word, it's one we should banish from our vocabulary. Not only are diets painful, annoying, difficult, and demeaning but they typically don't work forever. After all, no one can spend her entire life denying herself her favorite foods for the sake of calories.

So if you're looking for a calorie-counting, rice cake approach to weight loss, you'll have to go elsewhere. If, however, you're looking for a way to revolutionize your lifestyle to incorporate good health and healthy eating—with weight loss as a guaranteed by-product—then you've come to the right place.

Foolproof Weight Loss takes a deliberately holistic view of weight. It's not about pounds of flesh but about how we feel about ourselves and our lives, how we cope with stress and surprises, how we move through our days and nights. Most important, it's about learning to accept ourselves as we are—accentuating our inner and outer beauty, which have nothing to do with any number on a scale.

There is no quick fix to an unhealthy lifestyle, of course, so use this book as if it were a road map for your journey to good health. You can move along as quickly or as slowly as you like, taking what you need from each chapter and discarding the rest. In the end, any change you make will be a change for the better.

This book, like the other books in the Women's Edge health series, is jammed with the practical and doable—everything from how to dine in fancy restaurants and still eat right to how to transform your wardrobe to accentuate the very best things about yourself. We bust every excuse you've ever had about why you can't change, and we tell you how even the people you love the most can sabotage your efforts.

We do all this with help from dozens of experts and participants in the TOPS Club. TOPS, the acronym for the nonprofit group Take Pounds Off Sensibly, was founded in 1948 by a homemaker named Esther Manz. It's the oldest major weight control organization in the United States, and with 275,000 members, it's also one of the largest. Its basic philosophy is that to change behavior you need three things: motivation, skills, and support.

Foolproof Weight Loss will provide you with all three.

Anne Alexander
Editor-in-Chief
Prevention magazine

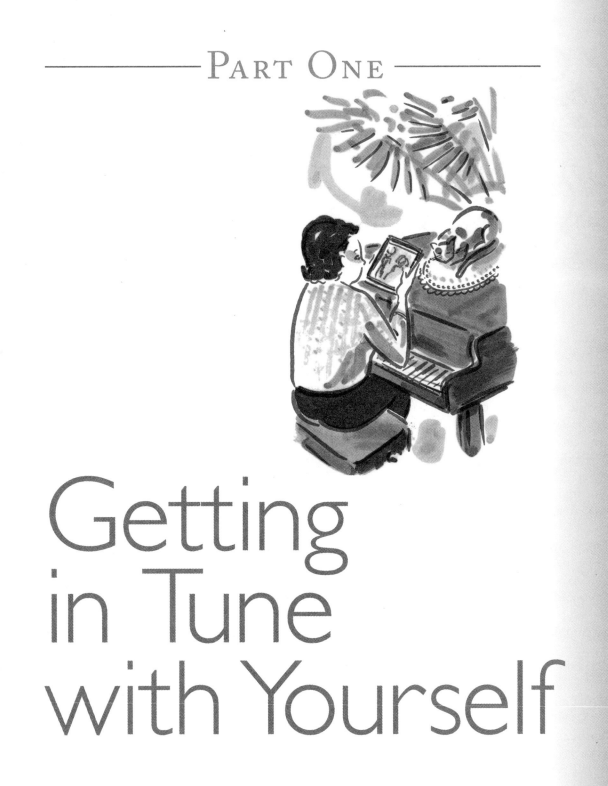

PART ONE

Getting in Tune with Yourself

Our Lips Are Sealed— Or Are They?

Any seasoned veteran of the fat wars can recite the basic formula for weight loss as fast as her phone number: Eat fewer calories than you burn. Still, we're always looking for a new twist. A new discovery. A magic formula to get the job done quickly.

Maybe that's why so many of us dive into diet after diet—on average, about twice a year—before we are ready to lose weight, and before we are prepared to make the permanent lifestyle changes essential to lasting weight loss success. As a result, we fail and fail again.

"Most people *think* they're ready to lose weight," says Sandra Haber, Ph.D., a New York City psychologist who specializes in women's weight issues. "Yet changing our health habits is a very complex, three-dimensional task, which has been foolishly simplified by standard diet formulas and remedies. The question should be: 'Are you *really* ready to lose weight?'"

Or, put another way, "Are you *really* ready to change?"

Research shows that permanent health-behavior change occurs in five specific stages, says Carol Boushey, Ph.D., assistant professor in

the department of foods and nutrition at Purdue University in West Lafayette, Indiana. Called the stages of change, the psychological model was first developed in the early 1990s to help people overcome high-risk behaviors such as smoking and alcohol abuse. Each stage represents a different mindset in the change process. It's now gaining widespread acceptance for use in helping people change behaviors related to diet and exercise.

Experts agree that if you can identify and understand the importance of each stage and how to use specific strategies that are effective in each, you'll dramatically boost your chances of progressing from stage to stage and achieving your goals. That's why short-term diets fail, says Dr. Boushey: They ignore your need to progress gradually through these stages.

It will take time. Some of us sail through each stage without a hitch. Others might think about starting an exercise program for years before actually lacing up a pair of sneakers. More common is the woman who makes several attempts at change before finally achieving her goals.

QUIZ: ARE YOU READY TO CHANGE?

Weight loss involves changing two areas of your life: the number of calories you take in and the number of calories you burn. Studies, however, show that less than one-fifth of us make the necessary changes in both areas when we set out to lose weight.

The fact is, you may be more ready to change your eating habits than your activity level or vice versa. Understanding your level of readiness allows you to develop your own personal strategy for mastering each stage of change. To find out which stage you're in, pick the answers that best describe your mindset right now.

Are you ready to eat right?

A healthy diet means eating at least five servings of fruits and vegetables, six servings of grains (some of those whole grains), two servings of lean meat or legumes, and at least two servings of calcium-rich low-fat or nonfat dairy products daily. It also means that you avoid or limit processed high-fat and high-sugar foods. And don't forget to include plenty of water.

1. I don't currently eat a healthy diet, and I don't plan to start.
2. I intend to adopt a healthy diet in the next 6 months.
3. I've started making some healthy changes to my diet.
4. I regularly eat a healthy diet, but I still have to fight off the temptation for high-fat, high-sugar foods now and then.
5. I have been eating a healthy diet for more than 6 months, and it has become second nature to me.

Are you ready to get moving?

"Physically active" means that your exertion level equals that of a brisk walk, climbing stairs, vacuuming, or digging in the garden, and that you accumulate at least 30 minutes of this level of activity 3 to 5 days a week.

1. I am not very active. I don't exercise, and I don't plan to start.
2. I've been thinking about becoming more active, but just can't get started.
3. I exercise once in a while, but could do more.
4. I've started exercising regularly, but it's still tough to keep up.
5. I've engaged in regular physical activity for more than 6 months, and it has become second nature to me.

Scoring

Note the number you picked and the stage in which you need to begin.

1. Precontemplation
2. Contemplation
3. Preparation
4. Action
5. Maintenance

In general, if you are thinking about changing a habit and are willing to make a serious attempt, you will probably spend a couple of months at each stage of change.

The first step in the process is to determine where you are—how ready you are to change your eating and activity habits. Once you've identified your own level of readiness, you can begin to build new skills that move you toward the permanent lifestyle changes that result in weight loss.

Precontemplation: Why Choose to Lose

Stage 1: You're not thinking about change at all.

In this stage, we're either unaware or uninterested in change, says Bess H. Marcus, Ph.D., associate professor of psychiatry and human behavior at the Brown University Center for Behavioral and Preventive Medicine in Providence, Rhode Island. She pioneered the use of stages of change to help people become more physically active.

Here, we don't see how losing weight will impact our lives. We could be in denial about the health risks of being overweight and inactive. Or, we could simply be worn down by repeated dieting failures. This is our comfort zone. We tend to stay at this stage for a long time—sometimes for life—because it feels safe and familiar.

A clue that we need to wake up may come from friends and family hinting that we need to lose weight, begin exercising, or otherwise change our lifestyle. Our goal is to stop tuning them out.

IS YOUR WEIGHT LOSS MIRED IN MYTH?

Over and over, we read that 95 percent of those who lose unwanted pounds gain it all back and then some, so why bother? Because that often-quoted statistic is a myth.

The 95 percent figure "has a toehold in our thinking, but it doesn't apply to most people," says Suzanne W. Dixon, R.D., a research epidemiologist and registered dietitian at the Henry Ford Health System in Detroit. The discouraging figure springs from one 1959 study of 100 people who were given a diet but no exercise or behavioral modification support. In the years following, Dixon says, a number of similar studies helped build a weight-regain mythology that remains today.

"The 95 percent figure has stuck, but what people don't realize is that these earlier studies were conducted among people in clinical programs, using last-ditch, extreme diets, like 800-calorie diets," Dixon relates. "These are people who were obese, not just overweight, their whole lives. Some had distinct medical issues and psychological problems with compulsive eating. They were the extreme end of people with weight problems, not the typical population who wants to lose weight."

So if the 95 percent regain figure is the stuff of weight loss legend, what percentage of people really *do* succeed at maintaining weight loss? As yet, there is no definitive answer.

Knowledge is power. Read, rent informative videos, or surf the Internet to gather health information. Consult your doctor, a registered dietitian, or a personal trainer. This process will open your conscious mind to the idea of change, says Dr. Boushey.

Discover the benefits. Even very modest weight loss—just 5 pounds—can improve how we feel and how our bodies function, according to a Harvard study of more than 40,000 women. Conversely, add too many pounds and you raise your risk of diabetes and heart disease. To quickly assess your degree of potential health

There is a project underway, though, that promises to replace the myth with a realistic number. The National Weight Control Registry (NWCR) is a database of successful weight losers created specifically to examine a large, general population that has maintained substantial weight loss. Operated by weight specialists from the University of Colorado at Boulder and the University of Pittsburgh, the NWCR is collecting information from those who have lost at least 30 pounds and maintained that loss for at least 1 year.

One of the more telling findings of the NWCR so far is that half the people enrolled have lost weight and kept it off on their own without any formal weight loss program or help. And, on average, those enrolled have lost more than 60 pounds and maintained a 30-pound weight loss for about 5 years.

"People who want to lose 20 or 30 pounds or even significantly more weight have real reason to use a positive approach," says Dixon. She notes that research indicates that those who are successful at weight loss have tried to lose weight several times before finally finding what worked for them. Then they continued to follow low-fat, moderate-calorie eating habits. One more thing: "They never quit exercising."

risk, calculate your waist-to-hip ratio. Simply measure your waist (1 inch below your navel) in inches and divide it by your hip measurement in inches. For women, a waist-to-hip ratio of 0.80 or more is associated with increased health risks.

Forget bad experiences. More than 90 percent of those in the National Weight Control Registry—a group of more than 800 people who have kept 30 pounds off for at least a year—tried to lose weight several times before they were successful. In fact, each had lost and regained an average of 270 pounds.

Instead of viewing previous weight loss attempts as failures, consider them a rich source of information of what has and hasn't worked for you in the past, says Dr. Haber. For instance, if eating three servings of fruit a day helped squelch your urge for sweets last time, but cutting out dessert entirely only induced binges, then go back to eating fruit and add a single serving of dessert two or three times a week.

Contemplation: The Wheels Are Turning

Stage 2: You recognize that there's a need to change, but you aren't quite ready to do anything about it.

The focus starts to shift inward, and we begin to evaluate our own behaviors and identify habits that we'd be willing to change. Our goal in this stage is to consciously make the decision to change. You'll know you're ready to move on when you're focusing on the solution and the future rather than on the problem and the past.

"There are a lot of changes to contemplate," explains Dr. Haber. "There are changes, for example, in how you set up your home, in what foods you keep in your fridge and pantry, and in the kind of meals you have."

This period of thought and reflection is crucial. Resist the temptation to skip ahead. "You're looking for reasons that will make changing important to you," says Dr. Boushey. "If you jump in too fast, you are going to fail because you are not ready yet." The length of time in each phase depends on the individual. Don't move to a higher stage until you've achieved maintenance in the previous stage.

Know your motives. Before you munch on your first carrot stick, evaluate your reasons for wanting to lose weight. Are you trying to please your spouse? Slimming down for a class reunion? Trying to lower your blood pressure? Or are you just trying to look and feel better?

"The decision to lose weight is strictly an individual matter. What works for one person doesn't necessarily work for another," says Kristi Ferguson, Ph.D, associate professor of community and behavioral health at the University of Iowa College of Public Health in Iowa City, who has explored whether our reasons for losing weight influence our chance of success. Researchers analyzed answers from 100 successful and 40 unsuccessful dieters and concluded that it doesn't really matter what your reason is for wanting to lose weight. What does matter is where that reason comes from. "We're more likely to succeed when our motivation comes from within—when we choose to lose weight for ourselves, not to please others," says Dr. Ferguson.

Before we can move beyond just thinking about losing weight to actually committing ourselves to a healthy lifestyle program, the positives of weight loss have to outweigh the negatives.

Think small changes. Lumping diet and exercise changes together as one giant goal is like trying to swallow a watermelon whole. A more manageable approach is to pinpoint individual habits or behaviors that you want to change, says Dr. Boushey. Each requires a different course of

WOMAN TO WOMAN

She Finally Lost Weight When She Was Ready to Change

Change has been a slow, steady process for Maura O'Connor, a 30-year-old sales representative from New York City. An avid exerciser, Maura has worked out at least five times a week ever since her college days. Yet she has always struggled to maintain a healthy weight because of poor eating habits. Then she met a nutritionist who was able to target specific habits that Maura needed to change. As a result, Maura has lost more than 20 pounds. Here's her story.

I was one of those fit and fat people. I've worked out consistently 6 or 7 days a week for the past 11 years. My eating was a different story. It fluctuated all the time. I'd join Weight Watchers and get my eating habits under control. I'd lose some weight, but then I would start overeating again. The weight would come back, plus some. Like a broken record, I kept replaying the same scenario over and over.

It was getting harder and harder to do the Weight Watchers routine, so I consulted a nutritionist. She outlined a 1,300-calorie-a-day eating plan for me and told me to start

research, planning, and action. For instance, instead of saying, "I'm going to eat less fat," you might decide to switch from whole milk to skim milk. "Set a goal that's realistic and doable that you can achieve in a short amount of time. Meet it, then pick a new goal," says Dr. Haber.

Recognize your barriers. Think of all the reasons why you haven't been able to lose weight in the past: "I don't have time to exercise. My family doesn't like diet food. Fresh fruits and vegetables cost more money." These are barriers—every reason we can think of *not* to change. To conquer our barriers, we have to learn the difference between an excuse (I don't have time to exercise) and the real reason (I don't want to get up early to work out), and find ways writing down everything I ate in a food diary. I wrote it down, but I didn't lose weight. I just wasn't ready to follow the plan she had outlined for me.

At some point, I decided that I wanted to look the way I felt. I wanted to look like the athlete that I am. Maybe it was because I was turning 30, and I realized that I was solely responsible for myself. Maybe it was a now-or-never kind of feeling. I guess I finally realized that I wanted to do this for me.

I started following the program that my nutritionist outlined and writing it all down. I probably spent about 30 minutes a day recording what I ate. The work and honesty paid off. I learned that my real issue with food was portion size. Gradually, I learned how much I could eat of everything. In 9 months, I've lost 20 pounds. Before, that would have seemed too slow for me. Now, I feel like time isn't an issue, because this isn't a diet.

My mind now works like a cash register when I'm tallying up portions. Keeping track of what I eat has become automatic. In fact, over the holidays, I was able to enjoy having a few cookies and treats just like everyone else, and still lose weight.

making small changes in your eating habits. You may even have a personal trainer, nutritionist, or program specialist to help you.

Once you have a detailed, solid plan of attack, you're good to go.

Plan a reasonable strategy. The key to successful weight control is choosing a plan and a lifestyle that is manageable and completely doable, says Howard J. Rankin, Ph.D., behavioral psychology advisor for the Take Off Pounds Sensibly (TOPS) Club and author of *7 Steps to Wellness*. You have to determine a realistic rate of weight loss. A moderately active woman who eats 1,200 calories a day may lose only 3 pounds a month. So she needs to accept that it may take her a year to lose 30 pounds. "There's no point in going to extremes to lose weight, because the chances are extremely high that you will put it all back on again when you *do* return to a manageable lifestyle," Dr. Rankin says.

to resolve those real reasons, explains Dr. Marcus.

Preparation: Map Your Route

Stage 3: You're ready, willing, and planning to change.

Now you have to figure out exactly how that's going to happen. "This is a good place to be. You can aggressively start to take action," says Dr. Boushey.

Once you move into preparation, change is no longer a far off, someday-I'll-do-that kind of goal. You're planning to dive in headfirst within the month. To test the waters, you'll probably start exercising once or twice a week and begin

Anticipate obstacles. Determine how you're going to deal with preset failure dates like Thanksgiving or vacation, or a trip to McDonald's, or when the nighttime munchies strike. "It's like going into war," says Dr. Haber. "You don't go into a war and leave your weapons at home. You go to war prepared."

Break it down. Even seemingly simple changes involve a whole series of steps if they're to work. Take fresh veggies, for example. You decide that instead of chips, you'll snack on carrots, celery, or bell peppers while you're watching TV. Great. But have you followed through to make this new behavior easy and appealing? Did you go to the grocery store to buy all the vegeta-

TOPS CLUB
AND WHAT IT MEANS TO YOU

Its name says it all: Take Off Pounds Sensibly. TOPS Club doesn't offer any quick fixes or phony guarantees. Losing weight is up to you. But while you're working on it, weekly TOPS chapter meetings can provide the encouragement you need to stick with your plan over the long haul.

"I believe that to change behavior, you really need three things: motivation, skills, and support," says Howard J. Rankin, Ph.D., behavioral psychology advisor to TOPS Club and author of 7 *Steps to Wellness*. "TOPS works because that's all it is—a support group."

A nonprofit group, TOPS was founded in 1948 by a homemaker named Esther Manz. It's the oldest major weight control organization in the United States, and with 275,000 members, it's also one of the largest.

Although TOPS endorses the basic dietary exchange program, your personal diet and exercise program is provided by your physician. TOPS provides lively meetings, motivational materials, and incentives to keep you going.

"People identify with the kinship and friendship that they find at TOPS," says Dr. Rankin. "It's called TOPS *Club*, and there is a certain element of feeling just like a club. That everyone there is struggling with the same problems is phenomenally powerful."

Like TOPS Club members, you need to take the safe, slow, sensible, and successful approach to weight loss. So throughout *Foolproof Weight Loss* you'll find inspirational and practical tips from TOPS members.

If you decide that you want to try out TOPS, finding a meeting close to home should be easy. There are more than 11,000 held each week all over the world. Your first meeting is free. If you decide to join, annual membership is just $20 in the United States and $25 in Canada. To learn more about TOPS, call (800) 932-8677 or check their Web site at www.tops.org.

bles? Are they washed and peeled? Did you cut them up into sticks? Do you have a low-fat dip to make them taste good?

"There is a fair amount of energy and effort, particularly in the beginning of creating a new habit, that is very unnatural and requires a great deal of willpower," says Dr. Haber. Eventually, stashing a ready-to-eat supply of sliced fresh vegetables in your fridge will become second nature.

Enlist support. If at all possible, surround yourself with people who are supportive or join a support group like TOPS or Weight Watchers. "Overall, you really do need support if you're going to change your lifestyle," says Dr. Rankin. "Unfortunately, it's an element of weight loss that is often overlooked." Support fulfills four important roles: It's a way of gathering information, getting encouragement, finding a facilitator, and keeping us anchored when we get off track.

Share your goals with friends and family. Show your spouse and other family members how they can help you, says Dr. Rankin. And keep in mind that some people in your life may actually hinder your efforts.

Action: Kick It into Gear

Stage 4: It's time to road test your plans.

You're psyched. You're ready. But to turn healthy eating and regular activity into lifelong habits, this stage requires a lot of determination and hard work.

Expect to encounter rough spots—situations where you're tempted to overeat and days when you'd rather have a root canal than break into a sweat. To avoid quitting before you get to stage 5, you'll need to develop multiple strategies for dealing with everyday obstacles.

For instance, if you know that you tend to eat under stress, have a list of alternatives that you can pull out when you feel like you're going to jump out of your skin. A bubble bath. A glass of wine. A nap. Maybe write in your journal or call your best friend to rant. Keep the list posted on the refrigerator so that it's the first thing you see when you reach for the cheesecake, suggests Dr. Marcus.

Remember these tips, too.

Give it time. New lifestyle habits are not developed overnight. "This is a major point to remember," says Dr. Haber. "You need time to focus on you, and you need time to practice your new eating and exercise habits."

How much time differs for every woman, but generally, 6 months of a new habit gives you enough time to build your confidence and your skills. By then, you'll have encountered your fair share of roadblocks along the way—bad weather, traveling, holidays—and found alternatives in order to stick with your new healthy habits.

Make adjustments. Even if you've planned your strategy carefully, you may be struggling. Regularly reassess whether your program suits you and whether it makes you feel good, suggests Dr. Haber. This may mean revisiting stage 3. "You're looking for a positive experience," she says. "The more you feel good about what you're doing, the more you'll look forward to it and keep it in your repertoire. The less you like it, the more quickly it's going to drop out and become a negative experience."

Bask in the rewards. Frequently, we forget to congratulate ourselves for our small successes—walking every day for a week, passing on the dessert during a romantic dinner, achieving a 5-pound weight loss even if you still have 15 more to go. "That's a little bit like climbing a mountain straight up and never stopping to rest and enjoy the scenery," says Dr. Haber. "Sit back and enjoy the view."

Also pay attention to the benefits of eating better and participating in regular activity, says Dr. Haber. If you have more energy, your clothes are fitting better, and people at work start commenting on how you look, it's sure to inspire you to stick with the program. And reward yourself occasionally for a job well done. Buy a new piece of clothing, get a manicure, or go to a movie (but skip the popcorn).

Be flexible. Slipping back into an all-or-nothing mode of thinking can trigger a relapse, says Dr. Marcus. Your plan to take a 1-hour walk at lunch evaporates when you get stuck taking a phone call at work. By the time you hang up, you have only 20 minutes to spare, so you figure, the heck with it. Wrong, says Dr. Marcus. Some exercise is always better than no exercise.

Maintenance: You've Got It Down

Stage 5: You're maintaining your new eating and exercise habits and are satisfied with the results.

If you've reached your weight loss goal, give yourself a well-deserved shopping spree. But don't stop now. To keep it going, use the skills you developed in earlier stages of change—focus on the benefits, reward yourself regularly, set goals, and vary your activities.

Mastering this stage requires patience and persistence and may take a year or more. A clue that you've truly progressed through all five stages of change: Your new lifestyle is automatic.

Expect to slip. Setbacks are a normal, natural part of the process. Your biggest challenges may be times of emotional and psychological distress—when you're bored, stressed, angry, or lonely. Unfortunately, these are the times when many of us use food to cope. If you slip up for a day or two, it doesn't mean you'll be back at square one, says Dr. Haber. "Pick yourself up, dust yourself off, and get going again," she says.

Learn to readjust. Since your new habits are ones that you'll have for life, you'll inevitably have new barriers to conquer, says Dr. Marcus. For example, your job changes and you can no longer exercise when it's light out. Or you move to a new city and have trouble locating a gym. Or your treadmill breaks. There are all kinds of situations that can occur. Don't let them send you back a stage or two.

Be supportive. Share what you've learned with other women you know who are trying to lose weight, says Dr. Haber. Helping others reach their goals is a good way to remind yourself of how far you've come.

Between the Devil and the Deep Blue Sea: Excuses

When it comes to weight loss, we can whip out a page of excuses longer than our weekend to-do list. And whine? Man, we can put a 2-year-old to shame whining about all the reasons why "now is just not a good time" to change our lives, our weight, our eating habits.

Intellectually, we know all the reasons why we should get on the weight loss bandwagon: Our cholesterol is too high, we can't stand the way we look, we're always tired and, oh yeah, we'd like to live to see our grandkids. Emotionally, though, we just don't want to do it.

So we make excuses as to why we shouldn't even start; that way, we don't have to do the hard work.

Often, what we think of as excuses are really solvable obstacles, says Karen Miller-Kovach, R.D., chief scientist for Weight Watchers International. "Excuses are artificial," she says. "As soon as one is removed, another and another and another takes its place. Whereas obstacles have solutions that can resolve the problem. The key is finding the solution that is acceptable to you. Otherwise, you won't keep at it for the long term."

And we're in this lifestyle change for, well, life.

With that in mind, here are some excuse busters from the experts—solid, simple-to-follow solutions that will dismantle your defenses and eradicate your excuses.

Excuse #1: Diets Don't Work for Me

That's true, and not just for you. It's true for everyone. Research proves what we instinctively know: Very little of the weight lost in diet programs is maintained over the long term.

"That's why you have to focus on lifestyle change," says Howard J. Rankin, Ph.D., behavioral psychology advisor for the TOPS Club and author of *7 Steps to Wellness*.

Excuse Busters

Integrate exercise and healthy eating into your everyday life. "Don't view them as something you're going to do until you lose the weight, after which time you'll go back to your 'normal' life," says Dr. Rankin.

TOP TOPS TIP

Without Excuses, She Feels Better Than She Did at 25

Peggy Malecha, 63, a TOPS communication ambassador and area captain for Arizona, has come a long way in the past 25 years. Back then, she weighed 225 pounds. Then her father died from vascular problems related to obesity, and her mother died from complications of diabetes, and she vowed to do something about her weight problems. She decided to start exercising.

Unfortunately, she hated exercising. She had a list of excuses: no time, exercise made her muscles ache, the gym was too far away, she hated sweating, she didn't want to wear shorts, she wasn't athletic enough, she was too old (at 35), and her knees hurt.

So how did she get herself moving? She added activity into her week slowly instead of jumping into an intense exercise routine.

She started out with low-impact aerobics twice a week. She went to a class once a week and did a video once a week. Gradually, she increased to three times a week, combining aerobics with walking. Finally, she joined a gym, where she began weight training and high-impact aerobics three times a week. With the strength training, she was able to get rid of her bad knees by strengthening her leg muscles. She realized that the more often she went, the more she enjoyed exercising and the quicker those excuses stopped slipping from her lips. Soon, exercising wasn't torture.

"Each time I lift a heavier weight and do aerobics a bit longer, it gives me a high," she says. "I may be worn out and tired at the end, but I feel great. I finally made up my mind that I wasn't going to be a fat person again. Like an alcoholic who can't drink anymore, I'm an obese person who can't overeat anymore. The biggest benefit of exercise is being able to maintain my weight while eating a lot of healthy food."

Today, she bench presses 50 pounds, leg presses 180 pounds, has more stamina than she did at 25, and doesn't feel any more pain in her knees.

Stop viewing weight loss as something that should be done *for you*. "As in, diets don't work *for* me," says Kristi Ferguson, Ph.D., associate professor of community and behavioral health at the University of Iowa College of Public Health in Iowa City. "This is something you have to want to do for yourself."

Go to the doctor. In one study examining what motivated women to start losing weight, a strong trigger was their doctors telling them that their weight was making them sick, or refusing to perform surgery unless they lost weight.

Focus on the positives. Like more sex. In one study of 32 overweight women, more than half said that their sex lives improved after they lost weight. They thought about sex more, had sex more often, or both because they felt better about their body image.

Excuse #2: My Metabolism Is Too Slow

"No matter how low your metabolism is, there's always something you can do to rev it up," says Dr. Rankin.

And forget the one about your metabolism slowing simply because of age. Some research indicates that most women put on about a pound a year between the ages of 30 and 40 not because of slowing metabolism but because of slowing up—eating more and moving less.

The less muscle mass we have, the slower our metabolism. And we do have to work harder as we get older to maintain that muscle. We lose about ½ pound of muscle a year during perimenopause and a pound a year during menopause. By age 55, if we're not increasing our activity level, that could equate to 15 pounds of muscle lost, meaning that we're burning 600 fewer calories per day.

Excuse Busters

Lift weights. Weight-bearing exercise builds muscle, which burns up to 25 percent more calories all day long, even when you're sleeping.

Eat frequently. No, not Entenmann's and McDonald's. But frequently eating small, high-fiber, low-fat meals that include some protein can keep your metabolism humming, says Dr. Rankin. "Every time you eat, your metabolism goes up. In fact, about 15 percent of the calories eaten are quickly used up in the process of food digestion."

Push past the set points. The irony here is that as we lose weight, our metabolism really does decrease, making it harder for us to lose, says Dr. Ferguson.

Upping your workout intensity or length, or changing the type of workout you're doing to challenge your body, can give you a boost, says Tammy T. Baker, R.D., an Arizona-based spokesperson for the American Dietetic Association.

Excuse #3: I Can't Afford to Join a Gym

So don't. They're expensive, loud, and filled with too many too-thin women in too-shiny spandex.

Excuse Busters

Work out at home. A University of Florida study of 49 women weighing an average of 190 pounds found that those who worked out at home lost more weight and did a better job of keeping it off than those who joined a group exercise program, like an aerobics class.

Swap. If you work out at home, you can replace the gym's Stairmaster with your teenager's bike, its treadmill with a pair of sneakers, and its weight machines with sets of lunges and crunches, followed by some lifting with a full water bottle in each hand.

Excuse #4: I'm Too Busy to Exercise

First of all, rid yourself of any preconceived notions about the word *exercise*. We're not talking a 45-minute run followed by a weight-machine circuit.

We're talking movement, integrating more activity into your daily life in ways that eventually will become so ingrained that you won't even realize you're doing them.

Simply increasing your normal activities of day-to-day living—fidgeting, moving around, changing your posture—can help prevent weight gain even if your calorie intake doesn't change.

Excuse Busters

Turn off the TV. We watch an average of 22 hours of television a week. And every hour of TV can be blamed for an extra ½ pound of weight per year. Can't give up the tube for exercise? Put your stationary bike or treadmill in the family room, plopped right in front of the TV.

Build it in at work. Let's start with e-mail. If you walked for 2 minutes to someone's office to deliver a message instead of spending 2 minutes at your desk typing an e-mail, you'd lose 1.1 pounds of fat a year. That's 11 pounds over a decade. Conversely, sit at your desk, and you're going to *gain* that 11 pounds. This "creeping obesity" is associated with significant increases in blood pressure, cholesterol levels, and insulin resistance.

So get up. Go to the bathroom on a different floor. Never take the elevator (unless you're on the 43rd floor, and then walk up at least 10 flights). Try push-ups against your desk and stomach clenches while you're checking aforementioned e-mail. Eventually, says Baker, you'll begin to see results.

Have a really clean house. We're talking the kind of clean that would satisfy even your mother-in-law. Vacuum every other day, including the furniture. Sweep the kitchen floor every night. Bend down and wipe those baseboards. Stretch up and clean the top of the refrigerator. Oh, and wear ankle weights while you're doing all this.

Pace while you're on the phone. Why do you think they invented portable phones? You should do at least $\frac{1}{4}$ mile around the house for every 15-minute conversation, says Baker. A quarter mile would be about 40 return trips to the end of an average-size room and back.

Act like a toddler. Watch how young children move, says Baker. They bounce around, climb the walls, and run from one room to the next with no purpose in mind. Ask them to bring you several things, and they're likely to bring them one at a time. "They're energy-inefficient, and that's what it takes to burn calories," she says. You can do the same thing. Carry items upstairs one at a time. Eat dinner in the dining room so that you burn more calories setting the

---

REAL-LIFE SCENARIO

She Can't Stop Joining the Feast

Sarah, 44, is a good mom to her two teenage boys. She makes certain that they're supplied with everything they need, from clothing to love, but what they seem to need most these days is food. She can spend hundreds of dollars on a typical trip to the supermarket, fill up her refrigerator and pantry, then see it all disappear within a week. She buys plenty of healthy items, including fruits, vegetables, and whole grain breads, but she also buys "boy snacks," which include lots of chips and cookies. The problem is that those "boy snacks" are never just for the boys. When the fruits and vegetables run out, she finds herself hitting the nachos right alongside her sons, but unlike them, she's putting on weight. What should she do?

Sarah already has one great habit: She buys fruits and vegetables to snack on. But, as she has probably already guessed, she simply can't eat as much of the high-fat and high-calorie foods as her sons. While the recommended calorie intake for 15- to 18-year-old boys is about 3,000 calories, a 25- to 50-year-old woman should be eating only 2,200.

---

table, carrying the food in, and clearing up. And stop asking your kids to bring you things; go get them yourself.

Get it in short bursts. Three 10-minute bursts of exercise throughout the day is just as effective at burning calories as one 30-minute set, says Baker. A 10-minute power walk burns 55 calories. Do that every day, and you'll lose close to 6 pounds in a year. You could break that 10 minutes down into even shorter increments. Waiting for the pasta water to boil? Drop and do 10 push-ups. Waiting for the pasta to cook? Add a set of lunges.

Avoid the drive-thru. Park and walk into the bank, dry cleaner, or restaurant. Even standing in line burns more calories than sitting in your car.

Luckily, she can use some snacking tricks to control her weight.

Since neither she nor her boys need the high-fat versions of snacks, she's better off buying low-fat varieties, such as pretzels or baked chips instead of those nachos she loves so much. If she does buy high-fat, choosing something she doesn't like, whether it's vanilla ice cream or salt-and-vinegar chips, will help her keep from indulging.

Since haphazard eating over the counter usually results in more calories, Sarah should set some snacking rules, such as eating only while she's sitting at the table. Once she sits down with a portion of the snack on her plate and eats it slowly, she'll probably eat less and still be satisfied.

Finally, Sarah can also start burning more calories, perhaps by walking while she's waiting for her kids' soccer practice to end or by taking an aerobics class.

Expert consulted
Nancy Cohen, R.D., Ph.D.
Professor of nutrition
University of Massachusetts
Amherst

Avoid machines. Instead of driving through the car wash, wash your car yourself (and wax it) to burn 306 calories in an hour. Use a rake instead of a leaf blower, a push mower instead of a gasoline- or electric-powered one. Throw away the remote control and burn an extra 3 calories every time your show ends and you have to (gasp!) get up and change the channel.

Excuse #5: I Am Too Stressed to Make These Kinds of Changes

You just lost your job. You're in the midst of a divorce. You're moving into a new house. Maybe my life is too stressful, you think.

Excuse Busters

Get real. "In reality, there's never going to be the ideal time to make these kinds of changes," says Dr. Rankin. "You can't expect life to stand still while you make changes."

Opt for a lifestyle change. Some studies show that it's not the major life traumas like divorce or losing your job that are most likely to result in physical symptoms, but those annoying, everyday occurrences like car trouble or running late for work that drive us to the antacids and aspirin.

Physical activity helps with that stress, and the activity doesn't have to be intense. In one study of 135 undergraduate university students, leisure-type physical activity like walking or riding a bike buffered the effects of stress more than intense aerobic activity like running.

Yet another study done by researchers at Duke University Medical Center in Durham, North Carolina, showed that the more physically fit a woman was—independent of regular exercise—the lower her blood pressure during a stressful day at work. This suggests that she's more able to remain calm during work-related stress.

Excuse #6: I Hate Cooking and Besides, I Don't Have Time to Cook Healthy Meals

"Cooking and good nutrition don't have to go hand in hand," says Baker. Nor does healthy eating mean that you can't use prepared or take-out foods as the cornerstone of your healthy diet.

GUILT-FREE PLEASURE
Aromatherapy

Think about how your heart flutters when you smell a newborn baby's head, or the warm feeling that washes over you when you walk into a house where someone is baking bread. There's a reason for those feelings: Scents affect our moods, says Barbara Close, president and founder of Naturopathica Holistic Health Spa in East Hampton, New York. It's easy to add aromatherapy to your life. Just follow your nose.

Choose your mood. You have no energy, but it's time for your walk. Stimulating scents include rosemary, peppermint, orange, grapefruit, and other citrus fruits.

Anxious and nervous? Soothe yourself with the calming scents of lavender, sandalwood, vetiver, myrrh, and frankincense.

Insist on authentic. Buy 100 percent pure essential oils—extracted from the leaves and fruit of the plant—over synthetic because the scents are stronger.

Use scents creatively. Light a scented candle, use a diffuser, or smooth scented lotion on your body. A couple of drops of an essential oil added to your humidifier will fill your room with scent for 2 hours. Mix several drops with an ounce of a carrier oil—almond, sunflower, or vegetable—and add it to your bath or hand it to your significant other for a massage (never apply essential oils to your skin undiluted). And don't forget to scent your office with potpourri or oils.

Excuse Busters

Buy packaged meals. Even packaged dinners like Hamburger Helper or pasta salad mixes can be healthy. Cut the oil they call for in half (you'll never miss it), substitute soy burger crumbles or low-fat ground turkey for hamburger meat and add in extra vegetables. In many cases, you can cut the calories by half and bring the fat down to nearly zero.

Do takeout. If Friday-night pizza is a staple at your house, don't change the routine, just the toppings. Instead of greasy pepperoni or sausage, order extra veggies and ask for half as much cheese on the pie. Or, pick up a rotisserie-roasted chicken at the deli, then add prewashed bagged salad and a 5-minute box of whole wheat couscous.

Buy prepared. More than half of us are buying those precut vegetables and prewashed salads. The reason? Convenience. So for a quick veggie to go with the take-out chicken, just dump some of those baby carrots into boiling water for 10 minutes and drain. Voilà! Instant vitamin A. Sure, the kids may grow up thinking that all carrots are 3 inches long and come in resealable bags, but so what? It's healthy and it's easy, and that should be our meal mantra.

Try frozen. It takes most fruits and veggies a week or more to reach store shelves, and then they may sit for days or longer before they hit your dinner table, losing valuable vitamins in the process. Frozen vegetables, however, have as many vitamins and minerals as most fresh, and sometimes more because they're frozen immediately after harvesting.

Buy canned. Then there are the divine gifts to dinnertime: diced canned tomatoes and fat-free refried beans. Drain and spread those tomatoes on a prepared pizza shell, top with already-shredded low-fat cheese, and call it dinner. Spread the refried beans on a whole wheat tortilla, add the same cheese and tomatoes, roll up, microwave for 1 minute, and again, you've got a healthy, easy dinner that even your kids will eat.

Excuse #7: I Can't Afford Healthy Food

Nearly half of us think that fruits, vegetables, fish, and other "healthy" foods cost more than the frozen french fries and corn chips that we've been tossing into the shopping cart. Well, check the prices. "Studies show that the closer foods are to their natural form, like produce, the less expensive they are compared with the prepackaged stuff we buy," says Baker.

For example, when researchers gave 300 people with high cholesterol information on cutting fat from their diets, those whose cholesterol levels dropped the most after 9 months cut an average of $1.10 a day from their food bills—a yearly savings of $1,600 for a family of four. That's enough for a massage every other week.

Excuse Busters

Shop smart. Buy produce in season. "It stands to reason that the strawberries shipped from Chile in January are going to cost more than the strawberries grown on the farm outside of town in May," says Baker.

Save more than just calories. Eating healthy can pad your wallet. You won't be buying high-calorie fast food and greasy snacks out of vending machines. "Plus, if you're healthy, you're more productive, and you have fewer medical bills," says Dr. Rankin. Not to mention the money saved on antacids and aspirin.

Excuse #8: I Hate Fruits and Vegetables

Oh, really? When's the last time you passed on the carrot cake or refused that double scoop of strawberry ice cream?

Eating fruits and vegetables doesn't have to mean substituting an apple for a piece of chocolate cake. Although raw fruits and veggies do pack the greatest amount of fiber and nutrients, nutritionists are happy if you get them any way you can.

Excuse Busters

Hide them. Try smoothies made with fruit, low-fat milk, and fat-free yogurt. Grate carrots into spaghetti sauce. Puree apples and pears with a pinch of sugar into luscious sauces for pork, chicken, or fish.

Don't ignore the obvious. Onions count. So does the garlic in your pasta sauce, the celery in your tuna salad, and the can of tomato juice you drank as a mid-morning snack. And what about that salsa you ate with your corn chips?

Go for sweet. Substitute dried fruit for candy. Just 2 tablespoons count as one fruit serving. Try dried cranberries, papaya, or cherries.

Puree them. Add them to soups, stews, and sauces. A word of warning, says Baker: Don't mix different-colored vegetables together if the sauce is supposed to add color to the dish. You'll end up with an unappetizing brown mess.

Excuse #9: I Absolutely Cannot Live without My Bowl of Ice Cream (Bag of Potato Chips, Order of French Fries, Etc.)

So don't. There should be no four-letter words used here (like d-e-n-y). "Just eat less of it, but don't give it up entirely," says Dr. Ferguson.

Excuse Busters

Try low-fat. But be careful. Don't double the quantity just because the fat is gone, says Baker. Low-fat isn't necessarily low-calorie, and it is calories that count in weight loss.

Try portion control. The minute you bring the grocery bags in, portion out your treats into manageable amounts. Scoop ice cream into single-serving containers and freeze. Divvy up potato chips into individual storage bags. Wrap cookies two at a time in foil and store in your pantry.

Excuse #10: I Eat Out Too Much (Especially at Fast-Food Restaurants)

Hey, even McDonald's understands that some of us are trying to eat healthfully. That's why most fast-food restaurants have selections that are relatively harmless in terms of fat and calories, like plain hamburgers (270 calories), salads with fat-free dressing (85 calories), and grilled chicken sandwiches (300 calories).

Other Excuse Busters

Order light. Restaurants now have to abide by strict government rules when they call something light. For example, low-fat foods can't have more than 3 grams of fat per standard serving. Menus must disclose why a light or "lite" food is light: Is it the color, taste, or calories? But be careful on the serving sizes. Most restaurant portions are two to three times the standard, meaning two to three times the calories.

Know your restaurants. Particularly if you tend to eat lunch out every day. Become familiar with restaurants around your office, then pick two or three healthy options at each. When you go, don't even look at the menu with its tempting descriptions and high-calorie, high-fat options. Just order your already-chosen selection.

Taste your food. Not sure if something is fat-filled? Pay attention to how it feels in your mouth. If it coats your teeth, the back of your mouth, or makes your lips feel slippery, chances are it's fattening.

Excuse #11: My Family Won't Eat the Healthy Stuff

Heard the one about the couple who was both eating a low-fat, nutritionally healthy diet? Only one of them knew it.

That's because there are many changes that you can sneak into your family's meals so gradually that by the time you tell them that steak-and-mashed potato dinner you just fixed is healthy, they'll think you've finally lost it. But they won't know that you chose the leanest cut of beef, cooked it so the fat drained off, used chicken broth instead of butter in the mashed potatoes, made that salsa with four different kinds of vegetables, and substituted applesauce for the vegetable oil in the dessert brownies.

Other Excuse Busters

Control portions. If your husband must have meat every night, then give him meat every night. But choose lean cuts of beef, poultry, and pork, and trim off every visible piece of fat. He may get 10 ounces. You should take only a 3-ounce serving, about the size of a deck of cards.

Add food. "You can generally sneak in one healthy food that you like at each meal," says Baker. "Make a lot of it so that you can eat a lot of it."

Watch the nibbles. "An awful lot of calories get consumed when you're preparing or cleaning up from a meal," Baker says. Before doing either, brush your teeth or chew a stick of gum.

Excuse #12: I'm Around My Kids (and Their Food) All Day

You have the hardest job in the world: You're a stay-at-home mom. And that means fetching 10,000 cups of juice a day, making 400 peanut butter and jelly sandwiches, and handing out at least 200 Popsicles. And, of course, kids never eat everything on their plates. That's where you come in.

Excuse Busters

Stop eating like a mom. This means throwing away the extra three chicken nuggets they didn't eat, scraping the ½ cup of macaroni and cheese into the garbage, and keeping your hands out of the Halloween candy.

Stop eating like a kid. If you're fixing them hot dogs and potato chips with sliced apples for lunch, fix yourself a turkey sandwich on whole wheat bread with lettuce and tomato, throw in some carrot sticks, and share the apples. If they're having plain pasta with butter for dinner, make yours with just a sprinkle of olive oil and load it up with steamed veggies.

Excuse #13: I Can Never Remember How Much I've Eaten during the Day

Given the warp speed at which you run your life, you're lucky you can remember your ATM password. Remember what you ate that morning? Please . . .

Excuse Busters

Write it down. In one study, those who were most consistent about writing down what they ate lost an average of 7 more pounds during the 6-week period between Thanksgiving and New Year's (the Bermuda triangle of weight

WOMEN ASK WHY

Why do I crave chocolate?

It's simple: It makes you feel good.

Look at when you have your cravings. Stressed? The sweet taste takes your mind away from that stress-causing problem. Hungry? Your blood sugar levels are low and the candy will raise them. Premenstrual? You're craving carbohydrates, which help increase the levels of certain feel-good hormones in your brain.

The bottom line is that chocolate simply satisfies us more than any other candy because of its mouth-watering combination of sugar and fat.

Most important, chocolate is associated with good memories from our childhoods: Chocolate birthday cakes, heart-shaped Valentine's boxes filled with chocolate creams, mini chocolate bars for Halloween. Maybe that's why chocolate soothes us more than apples when we're bored or stressed.

There would be nothing wrong with eating chocolate every day—if it weren't for our attitudes. We know that it's full of fat, so we tell ourselves that we can't eat it. And whenever we deny ourselves something, we want it more. Before we know it, the whole box is gone.

But if you allow yourself one piece a day, you'll do just fine. A mini chocolate bar has 36 calories and 2 grams of fat. Add it to your daily meal plan and subtract that pat of butter on the baked potato. Maybe the "craving" for chocolate will stop and the enjoyment will start.

Expert consulted
Connie Diekman, R.D.
Spokesperson
American Dietetic Association

loss) than those who didn't. In fact, those who didn't use a food diary ended up *gaining* 3 pounds.

Stock up. If you stock your pantry and fridge with only healthy foods—vegetables, fruits, beans, lean protein, whole wheat grains—then

WOMEN ASK WHY

Why do I get cranky when I'm hungry?

When you don't eat for several hours, your blood sugar drops low enough to stress your body. As a result, you feel light-headed, you have trouble concentrating, you get sleepy—and you may get irritable.

Whether or not you get to the cranky stage depends on how long since you last ate and what you last ate. Although we don't need to eat while we're sleeping, during the day, when we're burning more calories, we need to replenish our fuel stores constantly. We should eat 3 to 5 hours after meals and 2 to 3 hours after a snack. Grabbing a piece of hard candy or a can of soda doesn't do it—these simple carbohydrates cause your blood sugar to spike, but it's a temporary rise. Just as quickly, it plunges down, leaving you even hungrier, shakier, and more irritable.

To avoid those irritable feelings, eat some protein with every meal, like a lean turkey sandwich or beans, because protein is digested more slowly, keeping your blood sugar levels—and mood—on a more even keel.

Expert consulted
Claudia Plaisted, R.D.
Director of the nutrition and medicine
program
University of North Carolina
Chapel Hill

you won't have to worry as much about portions. Eat until you feel full.

Excuse #14: I Need to Lose So Much Weight, There's No Point in Even Starting

The weight you need to lose looms before you like a mountain. It's easier, you think, to just walk around it than try to scale it. But consider this: Even a mountain climber starts with just one step.

Excuse Buster

Start small. One pound at a time—that's how you put it on, and that's how you'll take it off and keep it off.

Excuse #15: I Just Had a Baby

The baby is out, but when you look at yourself in a full-length mirror, you don't see much difference between your reflection and a woman in her 6th month. All the more reason to get the weight off, but you can barely get yourself dressed by 5:00 P.M., let alone find time for a diet and exercise. Besides, you're up all night with the baby. Who has the energy?

Excuse Busters

Plan to breastfeed. Numerous studies show that it's best for the baby, resulting in fewer ear infections and allergies and optimal growth and development. But it's also great for you. You'll burn an extra 500 calories a day just feeding baby (calories you need to account for in your daily diet), and you have an enormous incentive to eat healthy, says Baker. But don't expect miracles. "Your body does hold on to fat when estrogen levels are high," she says, and levels are high just after delivery and when you're nursing.

Leave the house. Once life has settled down a bit and you're getting at least 4 consecutive hours of sleep, there's nothing better than putting baby in a stroller and taking you both for a walk, says Baker. "It's good for the baby to get out of the house and see new things and have new learning experiences."

Not only will you wind up retaining less baby weight but a study at the University of Michigan in Ann Arbor suggests that you'll also feel better about yourself overall and be more likely to do other fun things, like visit friends and family, pursue your hobbies, or go to the movies, than women who don't exercise.

Too cold or rainy to walk outside? Head for the mall—just leave the credit cards at home.

Excuse #16: I Just Quit Smoking

This is going to be tough, no doubt about it, says Miller-Kovach, since smoking typically consumes about 100 calories a day. But knowing this, you can resolve to eat 100 fewer calories a day or walk an extra mile per day (which burns 100 calories).

Excuse Buster

Exercise will help you stay smoke-free. A study at Brown University in Providence, Rhode Island, of 281 women showed that vigorous exercise actually helped them quit and stay smoke-free easier and longer than women who didn't exercise. The reason, the authors speculate, is because physical activity not only limits weight gain but also helps us handle stress better.

It Ain't Necessarily So: Weight Loss Myths

Every day seems to bring with it some new theory about what's to blame for weight gain. One day, it's genetics. The next, sugar and fat. Later, we hear that we should be eating nothing but protein, or maybe only carbohydrates.

If you're left confused—and frustrated—by all the contradictory information, join the crowd.

The reality is that much of the diet news we get is based on unproven scientific evidence. "Women should focus less on these news stories and much more on what they're eating and how much they're exercising on a daily basis," says Judith Wurtman, Ph.D., a nutrition research scientist at the Massachusetts Institute of Technology in Cambridge. "Then it won't make a difference what the latest diet fad is or what food is considered taboo, because it won't apply to them."

"Many diet myths are simply made-up theories that make it seem as though everyone is overweight for the same reasons. But we're not," says Denise Bruner, M.D., president of the American Society of Bariatric Physicians (a group of doctors specializing in weight loss treatments), who practices in Arlington, Virginia.

Some women are heavy because they nibble all day long. Others overeat only at mealtimes. Many never exercise. And some have true eating disorders, says Dr. Bruner. All these factors must be handled differently. "Weight gain isn't all about eating too much of any one particular food or substance," she says.

Here's the straight scoop on many common weight loss beliefs.

It's All in My Genes

The tendency toward large hips and thighs does run in families. And animal studies show that fat genes can affect how much we eat, our daily activity levels, and the speed of our metabolism. An unlucky few are born with slower metabolism than the rest of the world, but that's pretty rare.

"We've also learned that there are so many different fat genes that it would be impossible for people not to have at least some of them," says Teresa M. Gunn, Ph.D., a molecular genetics researcher at the Howard Hughes Medical Institute at Stanford University Medical Center.

But that doesn't necessarily mean you're doomed to be fat. In fact, only 40 percent of obesity is hereditary. The remaining 60 percent is a direct result of what you eat and how much physical activity you get.

And, while the number of obese Americans has risen dramatically over the past 20 years, with more than 50 percent of the population now considered overweight, we can't blame it on our genes because the gene pool doesn't change that quickly, says Suzanne W. Dixon, R.D., a research epidemiologist and registered dietitian at the Henry Ford Health System in Detroit.

What may be to blame is our lifestyle. We live in a high-tech society that keeps us sitting on our behinds in front of computer screens. We have drive-through banking, grocery delivery, automatic garage-door openers, and Internet shopping. Rather than cook healthy meals, we order in. Then there are the vending machines and fast-food restaurants on every corner.

We're simply taking in too many calories and not burning enough of them, says Dr. Bruner.

I've Reached My Set Point

Some experts believe that we're programmed from birth to be a certain size. This is known as the set-

WOMAN TO WOMAN

She Broke from Her Southern Family Tradition

As a child growing up in Greensboro, North Carolina, LaVonnia "Bonnie" Johnson, 46, often ate large southern-style breakfasts and down-home soul-food dinners. But after many years of such traditionally fat-laden food, the pounds piled on. Desperate to lose weight and preserve her health, she forced herself to break away from the southern cuisine and adopt healthier eating habits. Here's Bonnie's story.

I come from a family who always ate fried eggs, ham, bacon, sausage, grits, and toast with jelly and butter for breakfast. The eggs and grits were made in bacon grease. Dinner was fried pork chops, fried chicken, or fried fish. Even the vegetables were cooked in oil.

Unfortunately, I continued to eat like this well into adulthood. By the time I was 38, I was at my heaviest. I weighed 225 pounds and wore a size 22. What motivated me to get serious about losing weight were the frightening words of my doctor. He said that I would literally die if I didn't start eating right and exercising. I had high cholesterol and was on the verge of developing high blood pressure.

I came home one day and announced to my children that we were going to start eating low-fat and high-fiber meals. Right away, I started baking or broiling chicken and fish. I incorporated more fruits, vegetables, beans, and whole grains into my diet.

For breakfast, I now eat bagels, fruits, high-fiber cereals, or low-fat muffins. Lunch may include vegetarian salads, light Chinese shrimp dishes, tuna fish, or turkey sandwiches. For dinner, I may eat baked salmon, tuna, turkey chili, baked sweet potatoes, and lots of vegetables. Some days, my meals are strictly vegetarian. I also limit my sweets. Once in a while, I treat myself to a piece of pie or my favorite: butter pecan ice cream.

I've felt much better since changing my diet and beginning an exercise program. Now I'm an avid fitness enthusiast, going to the gym 5 or 6 days a week. Some days, my workout is cardiovascular exercise or weight training in the morning, followed up by a relaxing swim in the evening after work. Today, I'm 65 pounds lighter and counting. My energy level has increased while my weight and measurements have decreased.

point theory. According to this theory, our brains program our metabolism to speed up or slow down to maintain a set body weight, and there is nothing we can do to change that, says Dixon. So if we overeat, our metabolism burns more calories than usual, and if we eat less through dieting, our bodies burn fewer calories. This would mean that the lucky few will stay slender no matter how much they eat. For others, it means that they'll hold on to those extra pounds no matter how little they consume.

But while many experts acknowledge that metabolism varies among different people, there's actually no strong scientific evidence proving the set point exists.

"The idea that we're destined to be a certain weight, the set-point theory, is hotly debated by scientists," says Donna Ryan, M.D., an endocrinologist at Pennington Center in Baton Rouge, Louisiana. "Americans are fatter than ever before, not thinner, yet we have the same genes."

Weight loss experts are exploring the possibility that we may instead have a "settling point." In other words, once we reach a certain weight, our bodies want to stay right where they are, no matter what. That would explain why 60 percent of successful weight losers regain every pound lost within 2 years, and 90 percent gain the weight back within 5 years, says Dr. Ryan.

Food Is Addictive

One of our most enjoyable pastimes is eating. Food is the centerpiece at family gatherings, of-

WOMEN ASK WHY

Why is it harder to lose weight now that I'm in my forties?

Once you hit your forties, it's definitely easier to pack on the pounds than it is to take them off. With each passing decade, your metabolism (the rate at which you burn calories) gets slower and slower, mainly because you're less physically active than you were when you were in your twenties and thirties.

The second reason is that at this age you're probably in the throes of perimenopause, otherwise known as the change before the change. Your hormones are in a wild state of flux. As a result, they determine where and how much fat gets distributed on your body.

Then there's stress. Many women in their forties find themselves under a great deal of stress because of job and family pressures. The more stress you're under, the higher your risk for weight gain.

So what are the solutions? For starters, you must set aside some time for daily exercise. Ideally, you should get at least 30 minutes of cardiovascular activity followed by light weight training. Brisk walking, jogging, cycling, or step aerobics classes crank up your metabolism so that you burn fat and calories. Weight training kicks your fat-burning power into an even higher gear because it builds muscle mass. The more muscle you have, the more calories you burn—day and night. For every pound of muscle gained, you burn an extra 35 to 50 calories a day.

If you don't weight train, you'll lose, on average, about 5 pounds of muscle every 10 years up to age 40 and 7 to 10 pounds after age 40. That's 175 fewer calories a day that you'll burn each decade up to age 40. So by the time you hit

fice meetings, and parties. And it's a necessity we can't live without. So in a sense, aren't we all food addicts?

Not really. Food addiction is defined as an unhealthy preoccupation with food and an inability your forties, you're burning 350 fewer calories a day than you did when you were in your twenties. That's why it's not unusual to be 30 pounds heavier in your forties than you were in your twenties.

When it comes to your hormones, there isn't much you can do to whip them into their former twentysomething shape. By age 45, estrogen levels begin to drop, and that reshuffles your weight, your shape, and even the ratio of muscle mass to body fat. Estrogen in the perimenopausal woman (a woman in her forties to early fifties who still has her menstrual cycle) directs fat to the lower half of the body, namely, the hips, thighs, and butt. Eventually, it begins settling in the abdomen.

If you add some stress to the mix, you risk developing even more abdominal fat. Studies show that chronic stress causes your body to produce high levels of the hormone cortisol, which weakens your immune system and deposits fat deep inside your belly. That type of fat is implicated as a cause in diabetes, high blood pressure, heart disease, stroke, and possibly cancer.

The best stress relievers are aerobic exercise, weight training, yoga, meditation, and socializing. The key is to minimize the stressors in your life and insist on making time for yourself. If your job is a problem, find another one that's less demanding. If it's your husband and family, get help. That way, you won't feel so overwhelmed, and you'll avoid jeopardizing your health.

Expert consulted
Pamela Peeke, M.D.
Assistant clinical professor of medicine
University of Maryland
Bethesda
Author of Fight Fat after Forty

Some women use food for other reasons, such as a coping mechanism for dealing with stress. These women often have underlying psychological issues that they're not addressing, such as boredom, loneliness, and low self-esteem, says Dixon. "They need to address them if their food dependence is going to be resolved."

Diets Are the Best Way to Lose Weight

Contrary to what many women believe, extreme dieting is one of the worst things you can do if you want to lose weight and keep it off.. When we cut way back on calories, we rob our body of vital nutrients. That in itself sets off a complex chain of events that eventually slams the breaks on our metabolism. By not eating, our bodies literally think they're starving. So our fat-burning engines cool down and hang on to what fuel they have left. We may lose weight initially, but the pounds become harder and harder to drop as time goes on—in part because of nutritional deficiencies.

Here's the real kicker: Once we start eating again, it may take a while for our engines to heat back up. As a result, we may gain back the pounds we lost, and then some. "If you've been yo-yo dieting all of your life, chances are your metabolism is at its slowest," says Dr. Bruner. "It's your body's way of protecting itself from starving to death."

Diets are also fattening because they put us in a constant state of deprivation, which can lead to bingeing on our favorite high-fat foods. "The

to stop eating a particular food. It can take the form of emotional eating due to depression, anger, boredom, frustration, or exhaustion. And it can manifest itself as a compulsive eating disorder like bulimia or anorexia nervosa.

Women Ask Why

If I want to lose weight, will I have to eat foods that I don't like?

Not at all. Many women eager to shed unwanted pounds believe they can eat only cottage cheese, yogurt, fat-free milk, and fish. But that's not true. You don't have to give up eating roast pork and butter-drenched mashed potatoes completely.

Just identify the foods that you absolutely can't live without and try to fit them into your diet plan. You'll have to modify your recipes and make them less fattening, but there are lots of magazines and cookbooks that do that for you. Or, eat your favorite foods as they are but only in small quantities and on rare occasions.

A clever way to incorporate the lower-fat, healthier foods you need but don't really like is to make them a part of a larger recipe. For instance, if you don't like yogurt, make a cream of broccoli soup that calls for yogurt as an ingredient. Eat cottage cheese with your favorite fruit. Try Chinese vegetable dishes instead of the veggies you grew up on.

If you must have red meat, nix the burger and steak and opt for some beef-vegetable soup, beef stir-fry, or a beef stew made with carrots, broccoli, peas, onions, celery, and potatoes (white and sweet). That way, you'll scale back on the amount of meat you're eating while getting the vegetables you need.

Try to look at your weight loss goals as windows of opportunity to experiment with other types of low-fat, healthy foods such as Japanese noodle dishes or Thai and Vietnamese cuisine. Chances are you'll love these new choices and won't walk around feeling deprived.

Expert consulted
Judith Wurtman, Ph.D.
Nutrition research scientist
Massachusetts Institute of Technology
Cambridge

critical mistake that dieters make is that they eat very small portions and skip meals," says Dr. Ryan. "They'll forgo breakfast, drink a diet soda for lunch, and eat a low-calorie microwaveable dinner. They're starving. And when they do start eating again, they can't stop. So bingeing is really a physiological response to starvation."

I Need to Reduce Portion Sizes

Downsizing portion sizes at mealtimes can help you lose weight initially, but if you don't add regular exercise to the equation, you won't keep the pounds off. Why? Because there will always be days when you'll eat a few extra cookies or potato chips. The exercise will burn those excess calories to help you maintain your figure, says Dr. Bruner.

Fat Makes Me Fat

Packing 9 calories per gram compared with the 4 in carbohydrates and protein, fat can do the most damage to your figure if you eat too much of it. "But losing weight isn't just about calculating fat grams. It's about counting calories," says Dixon.

"There was a time when you could reduce your fat intake and lose weight, but with all the high-calorie processed foods now available, you often end up eating even more calories that get stored as fat," says Dr. Ryan.

I Can Eat All the Carbohydrates I Want and Still Lose Weight

Gram for gram, carbohydrates are lower in calories than fat. Vegetables, whole grains, and beans are great sources of complex carbohydrates, while most cereals, cookies, crackers, white bread, soda, and pretzels provide the simple carbs that we sometimes call starches and sugars. Foods such as fruits and potatoes fall somewhere in the middle because they contain both complex and simple carbohydrates. People forget that if you concentrate on complex carbohydrates, you end up eating fewer calories. As an added bonus, the fiber contained in complex carbohydrates will help fill you up and keep you full longer so you eat less.

"Carbohydrates are broken down into sugars. And if your body isn't using them, they will turn to fat," says Dr. Bruner. Ever since fat was labeled as the enemy, people started loading up on simple carbohydrates, not realizing that they were eating more food and exceeding the number of calories they needed, says Dixon. It doesn't matter if the calories are carbohydrate, protein, or fat.

Alcohol Is No Problem Because the Calories Aren't Stored

The evidence is mixed. Some studies show that alcohol causes weight gain; others suggest it doesn't, says Dr. Bruner.

But the reality is that your body doesn't distinguish between the calories from alcohol and those that come from food, says Dr. Wurtman. If your body doesn't use the calories from alcohol as energy, it will convert them into fat. Some research shows that alcohol drinking can actually lead to overeating. One reason is that when we drink, our willpower isn't as strong, so we may be unable to resist the temptation to overeat. If you're trying to drop a few pounds, it's wise to put down the wine glass during meals, says Dr. Wurtman.

Que Sera, Sera: Realities

At Boston's beloved Fenway Park, what people complained about most was not the antiquated restrooms or lack of skyboxes but, rather, the cramped seats. In a brand-new stadium planned for the city, fans will ease into bigger aisles and wider, comfier seating arrangements.

Detroit remedied a similar problem when it built its new Comerica Park and installed molded plastic seats that are 2 inches wider than the 17-inch wooden ones in the old Tiger Stadium.

And a Wisconsin company, Bemis Manufacturing, has come up with a king-size toilet seat it calls the Paramount, which is 20 percent larger than a regular one and comes in a special shape contoured to pamper people of all dimensions.

Regular size just doesn't fit our expanding proportions anymore. More than half of us are overweight these days, according to the Centers for Disease Control and Prevention. And the problem is getting worse every year. Between 1991 and 1998, the percentage of Americans who were obese (more than 30 percent above their ideal body weight) increased by 50 percent.

The question is: Why?

What Will Be, Will Be

Traditionally, society has always blamed fatness on the individual. We assume that we're overweight because of our own personal failings—we're undisciplined, lazy, gluttonous, and lacking in willpower. Well, guess what? It's not all our fault. Some of the factors that contribute to our being overweight are clearly out of our control. For example:

Genes. It's true that some women who struggle with their weight have their ancestors to thank. A family history of obesity increases your chances of becoming obese by about 25 to 30 percent. But heredity isn't destiny—your genes alone cannot make you overweight, says Michele Trankina, Ph.D., nutritional consultant and professor of biological sciences at St. Mary's University of San Antonio. What they can do is make you more susceptible to gaining weight by influencing metabolism, body type, appetite, and even how active you are from moment to moment—in other words, how much you fidget.

What's emerging from the raft of research is

that all of us simply have either a greater or lesser genetic tendency to gain weight. Tempting as it may be to blame your DNA, remember that it's only a small part of the equation.

Age. With age comes wisdom, laugh lines, and yes, a few more pounds. "It's not a matter of *if* we'll gain but, rather, *when* and how much we'll gain," says Linda Van Horn, R.D., Ph.D., professor in the department of preventive medicine at Northwestern University Medical School in Chicago. Research shows that, on average, women put on about a pound a year between ages 30 and 40. So that by the time we settle into our forties, about one-third of us weigh too much. And it doesn't stop there. The pounds continue to pile on. By the time we're through menopause, more than half of us are overweight.

The explanation is simple. As we age, we burn fewer calories, says Miriam Nelson, Ph.D., associate chief of the Human Physiology Laboratory at the Jean Mayer USDA Human Nutrition Research Center on Aging at Tufts University in Boston and author of *Strong Women Stay Slim.*

Each pound of muscle on our bodies burns from 35 to 50 calories a day; fat burns a measly 2 calories a day. Starting around age 40, most women lose about one-third of a pound of muscle a year and add at least that much fat, explains Dr. Nelson. As you approach menopause, these changes in body composition speed up. Lose 5 pounds of muscle, and you're burning 250 fewer calories a day.

GUILT-FREE PLEASURES
Massage

What tickles your senses more than a hot fudge sundae but doesn't add an ounce to your weight? A Swedish massage.

You may think of a massage as pure pampering—and that's not a bad thing. But it also offers some physical and psychological bonuses.

"Massage brings bloodflow to all the body's systems," says Mary Beth Packard, a registered massage therapist practicing in Ft. Worth, Texas. "When I'm teaching about massage, I like to start out with talking about bloodflow because that's the basis for everything."

The long, smooth strokes against the skin improve circulation and soothe the nervous system, explains Packard. The result: relief of muscle tension and stress. And stress, as we all know, can quickly sabotage any attempt at weight loss. "Massage is a good way to calm things down so that you may be less likely to overeat," she says.

Don't be surprised if you also notice that your skin glows and your digestion improves—two more key benefits of massage.

A massage is also a good way to feel more positive about your body image, even before you lose weight. "Very often, I have women tell me that they were apprehensive about coming in for a massage because they are overweight. But after one session, they're completely comfortable with it," says Packard. "Massage is a great body-awareness tool, a good way to get back in touch with your body."

Gender. Women are genetically endowed with more body fat and slower metabolisms than men. So, yes, it's easier for us to gain weight. "A woman's fat cells are physiologically different from a man's. They are larger, more active, and more resistant to dieting," says Debra Waterhouse, R.D., author of *Outsmarting the Midlife Fat Cell.*

Time of life. There are certain points in our lives where we're *programmed* to gain weight.

"The average woman has 30 billion fat cells," says Waterhouse. During puberty, pregnancy, and menopause, fat cells respond to increased and decreased estrogen levels by expanding and multiplying. In other words, we typically get fatter during the major hormonal shifts that occur with these life-altering events.

Our female fat cells also start acting a little more male during midlife. Instead of attaching themselves to our hips and thighs, they accumulate around the abdomen.

Society. As if maintaining a healthy weight wasn't difficult enough, simply living in America in the 21st century puts us at risk for weight gain, says Marion Nestle, Ph.D., professor and chairperson of the department of nutrition and food studies at New York University in New York City. We have access to a cornucopia of high-fat, high-calorie, good-tasting foods that are widely available, low in cost, and heavily promoted. "Food is an $800 billion industry in this country, and the objective of the food industry is to encourage people to eat more food, not less," says Dr. Nestle. The fact is, it's getting awfully hard *not* to be fat in our culture.

Consider these facts:

- Between 1970 and 1993, some 2,500 kinds of candy, gum, and snacks entered the market. During that same time period, about 1,500 new kinds of baked goods were introduced.
- Eight percent of Americans eat at McDonald's on any given day. The corporate

> ## THE STORY OF THE PIMAS: A TALE OF TWO LIFESTYLES
>
> In the Gila River Indian Community in Arizona, it's not unusual for a kindergartner to weigh 75 pounds. Or for an adult to weigh 300 pounds. More than two-thirds of the 11,000 Pima Indians who live there are obese. Among the adults, half have diabetes as a result of their being overweight. They are a community in crisis.
>
> Their genes are partly to blame. Like other groups of Native Americans, the Pimas may possess what scientists call a thrifty gene that encourages efficient energy storage during times of plenty to tide them over in times of famine. But there's more to the story.
>
> The Pimas settled as farmers in the Southwest nearly 2,000 years ago, establishing a sophisticated irrigation system in the desert that produced wheat, beans, squash, and cotton. Their lives were active, while their diets were high in fiber and very low in fat.
>
> Life changed drastically in 1890, when their water supply was diverted by European settlers. Starving and no longer able to farm, the Pima community had to rely on food provided by the federal government—mostly lard, sugar, and white flour.
>
> Today, the Pimas share the American culture. Sedentary office jobs have replaced farming and hunting, while fatty,

goal is to have no American more than 4 minutes from one of its restaurants. And that's only one fast-food chain.

- The average American child sees 20,000 30-second advertisements a year on television, and fast-food and food-product ads are ranked as the favorite among kids, so the food industry is obviously getting their attention.

But all this talk about food ignores the other side of the equation. Most of us are bulging not just because we consume too many calories but processed foods have crowded traditional dietary staples, such as cholla cactus buds and jackrabbit, off the table.

On the other hand, 500 miles south in the mountains of the Sierra Madre in Mexico, lives another Pima community of just 700 people whose ancestors separated from the main tribe nearly 1,000 years ago. On average, they are nearly 60 pounds lighter than their American cousins and six times less likely to develop diabetes.

The Mexican Pimas spend 23 hours a week in hard physical exercise, while the Arizonans spend less than 5. There are no labor-saving devices, not even electricity. They eat a traditional diet of fruits, vegetables, beans, and tortillas, all of which are high in fiber and low in animal fat.

For scientists, the striking physical difference between the two branches of the Pimas perfectly illustrates the impact of modern living on weight and health.

"The study of the Pimas provides strong evidence that lifestyle can win out over genetics," says Leslie Schulz, Ph.D., professor of health sciences at the University of Wisconsin–Madison.

Researchers think that if the Pimas return to a native diet and lifestyle, the risk of diabetes could be reduced. "The emphasis needs to be placed on cultural pride and retaining beneficial customs that are unique," says Dr. Schulz. But that hope may be unrealistic.

because we burn too few. From the electric can opener to the garage door opener, a century of labor-saving devices has necessitated the need for us to graft an artificial dose of exercise onto our days in order to stay slim.

Increasingly, weight loss experts are acknowledging the link between the environment in which we now live and how much weight we've gained in the past decade. It's unlikely that these changes are caused by lack of motivation or genetic or other biological changes in the population.

The Risk Factors You Control

In one survey, doctors and scientists involved in obesity research were asked to name the most important cause of weight gain. Their answer: genetics, a risk factor that we can't control. But in another study, researchers at Wesleyan University in Middletown, Connecticut, asked 3,400 people who actually were obese the very same questions and got some very different answers.

Both women and men believed that lack of exercise and enjoyment of eating were the most important reasons for their weight gain. "This was encouraging," says Ruth Striegel-Moore, Ph.D., professor of psychology at Wesleyan University and co-author of the study, "because it showed that overweight people were focusing on aspects of their lifestyle that they could change."

Regardless of our genes, age, or gender, the biggest risk factors involved in weight gain are lifestyle choices that we can control.

Here are some ways to take control of them in your own life.

Make muscles. Maintaining muscle is the single most important thing we can do to rev our metabolism and avoid middle-age spread, says Barbara Moore, Ph.D., president of Shape Up America! in Washington, D.C. Challenging your muscles for as little as 20 to 30 minutes twice a week with regular strength training can do the trick.

"We can increase our basal metabolic rate (the amount of calories we burn at rest) by 15 percent or more simply by building muscle," says Dr.

Nelson. One thing we need to be aware of is that our basal metabolic rate, or BMR, is responsible for about 75 percent of the calories we burn. And the single most important factor in determining BMR is how much lean tissue we have in our bodies.

Fill up with fiber. When we reach for the Snackwell's instead of the fruit, the pretzel sticks instead of the carrot sticks, or the cornflakes instead of the bran flakes, we're missing out on fiber. And a high-fiber diet, which is already linked to preventing heart disease and cancer, also may fight weight gain, according to a 10-year study of more than 2,900 young adults. On average, participants who ate at least 21 grams of fiber a day gained 8 pounds less over the 10-year period than people who ate the least amount of fiber.

"Fiber helps regulate appetite by making you feel full," says Dr. Van Horn, who co-authored the study. It also speeds food through your system so you absorb fewer calories.

Once known as roughage, fiber is found only in plant foods—fruits, vegetables, whole grains, legumes (beans, peas and lentils), nuts, and seeds. It's the part of the plant that we don't digest. The average American woman consumes less than half of the 25 to 30 grams that experts recommend.

Make time for you. Too busy to chop fresh vegetables, cook a healthy meal, eat a good breakfast, take a walk, or squeeze one more thing into your day? Maybe it's because you're putting your needs after everyone else's. "The biggest excuse I hear is, 'I don't have time.' I call it the type E personality—everything for everybody," says Dr. Trankina. "By the time we take

care of everyone else, we're exhausted." The daily time crunch is at the root of a lot of the risky behaviors that contribute to weight gain, from skipping meals to falling into the eat-whatever's-handy rut to sitting on the couch instead of stepping on the Stairmaster.

Focus on calories, not fat. "We think that by cutting fat, we can ignore calories. But you

REAL-LIFE SCENARIO
She Eats and Drinks to Her Heart's Content

Taylor, 37, has never been one to deny herself anything as far as eating is concerned. She has never really had to. When all her friends reached their thirties, they also reached for diet books. For them, the years seemed to have a way of adding pounds. But while they were going low-fat, Taylor could still sit down with a gallon of heavenly hash ice cream and never budge the scale. "Genetically blessed" was the way everyone described her. Her mother had been thin all her life, and so had her grandmother. She assumed that she would be, too. Now, she has noticed her clothes getting tight, especially in the waist. When she stepped on the scale after the holidays this year, she discovered that she'd gained 10 pounds. And her doctor told her that her cholesterol, triglycerides, and blood sugar were getting pretty high. Still, she's not worried. She's convinced that her genes will save her. Will they?

It's possible that Taylor is experiencing a change in metabolism that comes with aging. Our basal metabolic rates decrease by 2 percent per decade of life, all other factors being equal. Regular exercise can offset this decrease or at least make it less noticeable. Since Taylor doesn't do much in the way of exercise, she will most likely experience progressive weight gain as she gets older.

Her elevated lipids and high blood sugar indicate that she may be becoming insulin-resistant after years of eating anything she wanted, including an abundance of refined carbohydrates—sugary foods and high-fat foods. Insulin resistance is the inability of cells to recognize insulin, which is the key to getting the sugar called glucose into the cells. Consequently, the glucose stays outside the cells, elevating blood sugar, which can lead to type 2 diabetes. Taylor could have a glucose tolerance test done to obtain more information about her risk of developing diabetes.

She should consider cutting back on sugars and fats in her diet and beginning an exercise program that includes cross-training. This should include aerobic workouts, such as brisk walking or jogging, and strength training. This combination should result in higher HDL (good cholesterol) levels and lower LDL (bad cholesterol) levels. Taylor should also increase her intake of soluble fiber in the form of fruit, oat bran, oatmeal, and legumes (peas, beans, and lentils). A tablespoon of flax oil each day on salad or vegetables may also help lower lipid levels.

Another possible reason for Taylor's weight gain is hypothyroidism, decreased activity of the thyroid gland, which produces hormones that regulate normal growth and metabolism. It happens most often to women in their thirties, forties, or fifties. She should have a thyroid profile done to rule this out.

If Taylor continues to disregard the influence that her eating habits have on her health, she will surely be a candidate for lipid-lowering medications in the near future, type 2 diabetes and all of its complications, and possible cardiac bypass surgery in 20 years or less.

Expert consulted
Michele Trankina, Ph.D.
Nutritional consultant
Professor of biological sciences
St. Mary's University of San Antonio

10 fewer calories than the original version. Spread 2 tablespoons of low-fat peanut butter on a slice of bread, and you'll end up with only 10 fewer calories than the full-fat version.

But it doesn't end there. When our eyes see "low-fat," our brains say "eat more." To test how "low-fat" and "fat-free" labels affect food consumption, researchers at Pennsylvania State University in University Park gave 48 women three indistinguishable raspberry-flavored yogurts. When the women ate the yogurts labeled "low-fat," they consumed significantly more calories during the subsequent lunch and dinner than they did after eating the yogurt labeled "high-fat." When the yogurts weren't labeled for fat content, these differences didn't occur.

Move it all around. Nearly two-thirds of us are inactive by government standards, which means we get less than 2½ hours of activity each week. Whether we're sitting behind the wheel or parked in front of the television, physical inactivity is now built into our lives the same way strenuous labor was a natural part of daily life for our ancestors.

Today, the average woman expends about half the energy her that great-grandmother did each day. Our sedentary lifestyle is one of the main reasons why we're seeing a steady rise in the obesity rate, say a number of experts.

"We now know that most women aren't getting heavier because they're eating more," says Dr. Nelson. "The surprising reason that many women gain weight is that they're burning too few calories."

Ditch the diets. One out of every four

have to keep your eye on the prize," says Dr. Moore. "And the prize is calories." Consumption of fat declined from 37 percent of total calories in 1965 to 34 percent in 1991. At the same time, our calorie intake has climbed from 1,989 to 2,153 per day.

Low-fat often doesn't equal low-cal. Eat a fat-free fig cookie, and you'll actually consume only

<u>YOU ARE WHAT YOU DRINK:</u>
<u>BEVERAGES LINKED TO WEIGHT GAIN</u>

We may be gaining weight because of what we drink, not what we eat. Researchers at Purdue University in West Lafayette, Indiana, found that when people consume solid foods, they compensate for those calories by eating less of other foods. When they consume beverages, however, total calorie intake goes up, and so does their weight.

Americans are drinking more caloric beverages than ever before. Since the 1970s, soda consumption has more than doubled. We're drinking more of it than coffee, tea, and juice combined. In fact, one out of every four beverages consumed in the United States is a soft drink, according to the National Soft Drink Association in Washington, D.C. This averages out to about 56 gallons of the sugary stuff per person per year—a mind-boggling 85,263 calories a year, or about 245 extra calories a day.

Skip the soda, and instead drink eight 8-ounce glasses of water a day, says Denise Bruner, M.D., president of the American Society of Bariatric Physicians, who practices in Arlington, Virginia. Besides having zero calories, water naturally suppresses your appetite by filling you up so that you eat less. It also helps your body metabolize stored fat and clear your system of wastes.

Dr. Bruner has her patients fill a bottle or pitcher with their daily water allotment and keep it on their desks at work or on the kitchen table at home. "You need to make a pact with yourself that you're not going to go home until you finish those cups," she says.

tiply even further, says Waterhouse. Fat cells evolved to take care of us during times of famine—or calorie restriction—by holding on to the fat we have and becoming more aggressive at taking in new fat once the diet is over.

What's more, rationing your calories too stringently triggers hormonal shifts that help your body conserve calories instead of burning them. And at least 25 to 30 percent of the weight we lose by dieting is water, muscle, bone, and other lean tissue—not fat. The faster you lose weight, the more lean tissue you lose.

All of this points to a slower metabolism. In fact, the wrong diet can reduce your metabolic rate by up to 30 percent.

Eat where you sleep. The increase in obesity closely follows the trend of eating away from home more often, says Dr. Nestle. "The more we eat out, the more we eat, and the fatter we get."

It's no wonder. A typical restaurant meal *without* an appetizer or dessert contains 1,000 calories. A study of 129 women found that those who ate out the most—more than six times per week—consumed an average of 300 more calories a day than women who ate out less often. The extra calories, which came primarily from fat, didn't add up to extra nutrition either, notes Linda Eck Clemens, R.D., Ed.D., professor of clinical nutrition at the University of Memphis, who led the study.

Think small. When was the last time your

Americans is currently dieting, according to the Calorie Control Council. Most middle-age women have been on at least 15 diets since their teenage years. You'd think with all this dieting that we'd be getting thin. But we're not, because diets are fattening.

Diets boost the ability of our fat cells to store fat, to take in new fat, and in some cases, to mulfamily got seven servings from a 7-ounce bag of chips? From supersize fast-food fries to a movie theater box of chocolates, we tend to eat more when we buy large sizes, says Dr. Nestle. People will often eat 25 to 50 percent more—especially pure-pleasure foods like candy, chips, and buttered popcorn—when they come in bigger sizes.

"We buy large sizes because we perceive them as a good value," says Dr. Nestle. But we've lost our sense of exactly how big one portion should be. One hundred students taking a nutrition course were asked to bring in a bagel, baked potato, muffin, or cookie that they considered "medium." Then they compared those foods with the serving sizes that the USDA considers medium. Here are the results.

- A typical medium baked potato was 7 ounces, instead of the USDA's 4 ounces.
- A typical medium bagel was 4 ounces, double the USDA's 2 ounces.
- A typical medium muffin was 6 ounces, triple the USDA's 2 ounces.

It's not enough to make smart choices about what you're eating. You also have to pay attention to how much.

Write it down. When it comes to remembering what we've eaten during the day, a lot of us develop a case of food amnesia. So keeping a food journal can be helpful. "We get busy and tend to forget what we've eaten," says Denise Bruner, M.D., president of the American Society of Bariatric Physicians (a group of doctors who specialize in weight loss treatments), who practices in Arlington, Virginia. And without an awareness of what you've actually consumed, the calories can add up before we can say double cheeseburger.

Lady Be Good: Following Fads

Alice isn't stashing pretzels in her pantry anymore—or anything else that's low-fat, for that matter. In fact, so far today, she has eaten steak and eggs for breakfast, pork rinds for a snack, sliced ham for lunch, more pork rinds in the afternoon, ground beef patties for dinner, and now . . . She stares at that bag of shriveled, gnarly strips of pig skin and doesn't know if she can stand to put one more into her mouth. Maybe she should run out to the market for some hot dogs or chicken wings. This way of losing weight isn't turning out to be as much fun as she thought it would.

Alice is well-versed on the weight-gaining consequences of eating fat. She can even rattle off exactly how many grams of the greasy stuff you'd consume in a handful of Hershey Reese's Pieces (10 grams), a tablespoon of regular salad dressing (7 grams), or a cheeseburger with fries (36 grams).

But despite her ever-expanding font of nutrition know-how, Alice just hasn't managed to drop those 20 pounds that have been standing between her and a pair of size 10 jeans for years. So every now and then, she finds a brand-new fad diet bandwagon to jump on.

Which is how she came to be here, at her kitchen table at nine o'clock in the evening, facing down a bag of pork rinds. She never thought she'd be willing to kill for a nice fresh tossed salad or a plain baked potato, but that's how she's feeling right now.

Like the Ghost of Fad Diets Past, the hunger gnawing at her stomach seems to bring back visions of all her previous frustrating attempts to lose weight: Her run for the Kaopectate after eating nothing but grapes for an entire day on a Hollywood-style diet. Choking down a glass of an energy-boosting, muscle-building liquid protein supplement on an empty stomach. And what *was* she thinking when she bought that mysterious fat-burning spray for $29.95, plus shipping, that promised to blast away unwanted pounds and inches an instant after she sprayed it into her mouth?

She figures she has lost and gained the same 10 to 20 pounds at least eight times. But she dreads the thought of remaining in the oversized sweatsuit brigade.

So she's hanging her hopes on yet another diet—one more grab at that brass ring fantasy of a slinky, sylph-like new self. This time around, she's zapping the fat with a high-protein, low-carbohydrate regimen. If it worked for Aunt Helen, it can work for her.

Of course, there are trade-offs to consider. Just thinking about Aunt Helen's stinky breath that smells kind of like nail polish remover—a side effect of the diet—makes Alice queasy.

She leaps up from the table and throws open the pantry door. There it is: a box of linguine. She knows she shouldn't eat it, but she doesn't know if she can resist. She tears open the package . . .

The Problem with Fad Diets

According to a government survey, nearly 44 percent of us are trying to lose weight. The problem is how we're going about it. Of those who diet, only one-fifth are doing it the right way—by eating fewer calories and getting at least 2½ hours of physical activity a week. The rest of us, like Alice, are doing it the wrong way.

That comes as no surprise. We all know how monotonous it can be to monitor our intake and measure portions. And sometimes we get just plain worn out from trying so hard. So it's easy to see why we're tempted by information that promises a quick fix.

Not only that, but many of us probably *will* lose weight on the average fabulous fad for a very simple reason: We're eating fewer calories. No matter what regimen they prescribe, most fads simply restrict calorie intake in one way or another. So what's wrong with them, anyway?

You can't stay on them. Because fad diets require drastic changes in your eating patterns, you just can't stay on them for long. "Fad diets usually last about a week. By week two, you're usually on the downside of the diet," says Melinda Manore, R.D., Ph.D., professor of nutrition at Arizona State University in Tempe.

THE FIRST DIET

Question: In 1880, if you refused an offer for a slice of apple pie because you were watching your weight, you would have said, "No thanks, I'm _____."

A. Dieting

B. Reducing

C. Banting

D. Torturing myself

The answer is C. The first modern-day diet wasn't called a diet. It was called banting, named for William Banting, a fashionable London undertaker who had lost more than 50 pounds. By the age of 65, Banting was so large that he could not tie his own shoes and had to walk down the stairs backward. Excess tissue in his throat pressed on his eustachian tubes and impaired his hearing.

His doctor prescribed a diet free of starch and sugar. Banting did so well on the diet of lean meat, dry toast, soft-boiled eggs and green vegetables that by the following year, he was down to a trim 150 pounds and could walk down the stairs forward. His hearing had also returned.

Wanting to share his good news, Banting wrote up and printed 2,500 copies of his *Letter on Corpulence*. By the time he died in 1878, more than 58,000 copies of his diet book had been sold, and *banting* had become the new lingo for reducing.

Remember those pork rinds? Dr. Manore admits that she tried her share of fad diets before she became a nutritionist.

In college, she went on a high-protein diet with her roommate. Since they didn't have a kitchen in their dorm room, the pair decided that their protein sources would be Vienna sausages and Kentucky Fried Chicken. For a week, they ate nothing except canned mini-wieners and cold fried chicken. And they lost weight. Her resolve vanished when she visited a friend who had just baked an apple pie. "I called my roommate and said, 'I don't care what you do, but I'm having a piece of pie.' And the diet was over," recalls Dr. Manore. She had lost 5 pounds, but by the next day, 3 of them had already come back.

You're more likely to gain it back. Fad diets don't teach good nutrition habits, which means that once the diet is over, most of the weight is regained, explains Dr. Manore. "The dieter learns nothing about good food choices or making long-term changes in diet and exercise habits." The result is that once you go off the diet, you slip back into your old habits—the same ones that caused you to gain weight in the first place.

You keep the fat and lose your muscle. When we talk about wanting to lose weight, what we really mean is that we want to lose fat. Well, that's not what you get on most fad diets, especially high-protein, no-carbohydrate plans, says Dr. Manore. The plunging needle on the scale isn't telling you what's going on *inside* your body.

Most of the weight lost on a no-carb diet is water. Here's why: Carbohydrates are our primary source of energy. And our bodies are able

THE HAWAIIAN DIET: A BACK-TO-BASICS APPROACH

Too often, we turn to science for answers, especially when it comes to losing weight. We await the next big discovery, hoping that it will unlock the secret to shedding pounds quickly and easily. Native Hawaiians are taking a back-to-basics approach to combat a statewide obesity epidemic.

They're turning to the traditional foods that their ancestors thrived on—taro, sweet potatoes, breadfruit, bananas, and steamed fish—to lose weight and regain their health. The traditional Hawaiian diet is low in total fat (about 10 percent), high in complex carbohydrates (78 percent), and high in total fiber (30 grams per day), and it contains an adequate amount of protein and minerals.

"This diet is what the Hawaiians practiced for centuries before Captain Cook's arrival," says Claire Hughes, R.D., Dr. P.H., chief of the health, promotion, and education branch of the Hawaii State Department of Health. "What's more, these basics embrace cultural values and beliefs around the foods that were familiar to their parents and grandparents. The resurgence of the belief system that supports healthy eating practices makes a lot of sense to native Hawaiians."

to store only a limited amount of this energy in the liver and muscle tissue—about 1,000 grams. For each gram of carbohydrate stored, we also store 4 grams of water. These water reserves are there to help us cool down when we exercise by producing sweat. When we restrict carbohydrate intake, our energy-starved bodies tap into those stored carbs. We find ourselves making more trips to the bathroom as our bodies get rid of all the water that was stored along with those carbs. And violà! Weight loss.

We may feel pretty happy when we look at the scale and see a 6-pound loss after just a week of dieting. But less than a third of that weight

Obesity rates there have spiraled since the 1980s, as they have on the mainland. The problem, however, is worse among native Hawaiians. About 50 percent are overweight or obese, compared with about 28 percent of the overall population. With the increasing obesity rate has come increasing rates of heart disease, diabetes, and other chronic illnesses.

"Captain Cook found healthy natives living here," explains Dr. Hughes. As the islands became more Westernized in the mid-20th century, so did the diet of its people. Land development closed taro farms, fish ponds, and other food production areas that had been maintained by natives for centuries.

The Traditional Hawaiian Diet is a 3-week program conducted in groups of 25 to 30 people. Participants come to a community site for three meals a day prepared with traditional foods. One or two new vegetables are introduced each day. In all the programs, the overall health of the participants increased dramatically in addition to their losing weight.

While these community diet programs usually run for 3 weeks, Dr. Hughes stresses that the traditional Hawaiian diet is promoted as a lifelong program.

will be fat. You can double fat loss if you simply have a little patience and stick with a traditional low-calorie diet, says Dr. Manore.

They lack the essentials. Fad diets often eliminate whole food groups that provide essential nutrients, energy, and fiber. This isn't usually a problem since you can't stay on them long enough to develop a nutritional deficiency. Even so, it's a good idea to take a daily multivitamin supplement if you're dieting, says Dr. Manore. "Most dieters cannot meet the recommended vitamin and mineral requirements if they're consuming fewer than 1,200 to 1,600 calories a day," she says.

Most fads don't encourage physical activity. Fad diets almost never address the issue of exercise, yet it's an indispensable part of the healthy weight loss equation. "After all these years, I'm convinced that exercise is the key to maintaining lean tissue when you're dieting. It's also the key to maintaining weight loss," says Dr. Manore. Ironically, when you're on a very low calorie fad diet, moving around is more difficult. Rigid diets often don't provide enough carbohydrate calories to fuel our brains or recharge our muscles. The result is that we feel like we need a dose of Geritol.

They can be bad for your health. Protein-rich diets tend to be chock-full of saturated fat and cholesterol, which can increase the risk of heart disease. When carb calories are drastically reduced, the body starts converting fatty acids into a fuel that the brain can use, since not enough glucose is being provided by the diet. These release chemicals into the bloodstream called ketones that can cause headaches, dizziness, fatigue, nausea, and bad breath. Too much protein can also tax the kidneys, which go into overdrive trying to process and excrete high levels of nitrogen and protein, explains Dr. Manore.

Sorting Fact from Fiction

Like lottery tickets and slot machines, fad diets appeal to our desire for an easy way out. We want to be thin and we want it now. This may explain why Americans plunk down $33 billion every year for weight loss products and plans—much of it gimmicks that simply don't work. Before you spend your hard-earned cash,

WOMAN TO WOMAN
She Tried the Protein Diet

With her wedding only months away, Jennifer Turnbull, a hospital admissions clerk in Columbia, South Carolina, did what a lot of brides-to-be do: She went on a diet. To lose a lot of weight as fast as possible, she decided to try the popular high-protein, low-carbohydrate Atkins Diet. She expected to get thin and ended up in the hospital instead. The worst part? Every pound she lost returned, and then some. Here's her story.

I wanted to lose a lot of weight fast, so I went on the Atkins Diet. I felt great at first. I had lots of energy. I was on that euphoric high that you experience when you first start a diet. In just 3 to 4 weeks, I'd lost 17 or 18 pounds.

I faithfully followed the plan. My typical breakfast was eggs and sausage or bacon or ham. No grits. No cereal. No juices. I ate a ton of cheese. For dinner, I would have steak and some green vegetables with butter. Even though I'm a noodle nut, I didn't really feel hungry or deprived.

But I noticed after the second week that I had no stamina. When I exercised, I literally felt physically drained. It was the worst feeling, but I continued exercising regardless. But without carbohydrates, my body had no energy. Then one day, I passed out at the gym. The next day, I went to my doctor, and she rushed me to the hospital. She said I was dehydrated. My doctor kept me in the hospital overnight and put me on intravenous fluids. She also said to go off the diet.

As soon as I started eating like a normal person again, it didn't take long to gain back the 17 pounds I'd lost, and then 8 more. I was worse off than when I'd started the diet.

I know that the diet has worked for a lot of people, but it's not for everybody, especially people who need to lose a lot of weight. How long can you go without eating basic staples like rice, noodles, and bread? Can you live like that forever? These days, I'm taking the slow, sensible approach to managing my weight. I eat healthy foods and watch my portions. I walk at least 2 miles a day just getting to and from my car at the hospital where I work.

It's been about 2 years since I went on the Atkins Diet, and you know, I still can't stand to eat cheese after I ate so much of it for those few weeks.

learn to recognize some common weight loss come-ons.

The miracle food diet. When it debuted in the 1930s, the Hollywood Diet called for a few select vegetables, a small amount of protein, and lots of grapefruit, which was believed to contain a special fat-burning enzyme. The idea that grapefruit could speed up weight loss caught on and over the years spawned more than a dozen different diets starring the large, sometimes bitter, citrus fruit.

Sure, grapefruit is fat-free, low in calories, and packed with vitamin C. Its high fiber and water content help fill you up. But does it stoke up your fat-burning furnace? Not a chance. "Foods don't burn fat. They create fat when we eat more calories than our bodies need," says Audrey Cross, Ph.D., nutrition professor at the Institute of Human Nutrition at Columbia University in New York City.

The all-you-can-eat diet. The soup du jour served at this all-you-can-eat buffet is stewed from a head of cabbage, flavored with onions, celery, green peppers, and a packet of onion soup. You can spoon up as much as you want for 7 days on the cabbage soup diet, which falsely claims that it is a healthy way for heart patients lose up to 17 pounds prior to surgery.

The bottom line is that any diet that calls for bizarre quantities of one type of food—whether it's cabbage soup, rice, or steak—violates the first basic principle of good nutrition: to balance your diet with a variety of foods, says Dr. Cross. Diets like these are so boring that you simply end up eating fewer calories.

The nutrients-are-bad diet. Beware of fad diets that resemble a Saturday-morning cartoon, with one nutrient pitted against another. Instead of Superman, Batman, and Wonder Woman, the cast of starring characters are protein, carbohydrates, fat, and (on rare occasions) alcohol—the four sources of calories in our diet. The scenario usually goes something like this: Nutrient A is the cause of all your weighty woes. Nutrient B is the solution to your troubles. A dietary version of the old blame game.

"We love to buy into this idea that there's something metabolically wrong with us that a certain combination of foods can fix," says Dr. Manore.

Since the mid-1980s, we've seen fat typecast as our nutritional arch villain. If you wanted to be thin, a low-fat diet was your ticket. You could eat what you wanted, as long as it didn't have fat. But it turned out that all the fat-free food we loaded up on was still chock-full of calories and only made us fatter.

In the backlash, carbs became the new dietary no-no, fueling a flurry of fresh fads with names like Sugar Busters!, Protein Power, The Carbohydrate Addict's Diet, and Dr. Atkins' New Diet Revolution. All of these diets cast protein as the new nutritional superhero and fat as its friendly sidekick.

And so it goes. The cycle repeats itself over and over. Fat, protein, carbohydrate—who will be the bad guy next?

Top TOPS Tip

She Gave Up On Fads and Finally Lost Weight

According to her calculations, Barbara Cady, 56, a former college instructor from Fairmont, West Virginia, who first joined TOPS in 1964, lost and gained about 900 pounds on fad diets over the past 35 years. "If there was a book on it, I tried it," she says.

Most things worked short term, but never for the long term, Cady discovered. When she finally gave up on the quick-fix approach for good, she was able to come up with a plan that she could live with for life, and she lost 47 pounds. Here's her advice.

Forget about prescribed diets and stick with a balance of foods you enjoy. The trick is simply to eat less of them. "Weight loss is a journey. And it's essential that you enjoy that journey if you're going to stick with it to the end," says Cady.

She found a way to enjoy her favorite—pizza—and still lose weight. Instead of ordering a thick crust, Barbara now orders thin crust. Then she tops it with loads of veggies and maybe a little Canadian bacon and skips the pepperoni and sausage.

"I finally connected all the dots in the picture. I understand now that weight control is not just about one thing. It's about all things," she says.

The rapid-weight-loss diet. *Lose 30 pounds in 30 days.* Maybe you have seen this claim or one similar to it and been tempted to try it out. This is a classic case of "if it sounds too good to be true, it probably isn't true," says Denise Bruner, M.D., president of the American Society of Bariatric Physicians (a group of doctors who specialize in weight loss treatments) and a physician practicing in Arlington, Virginia.

The truth is that it's physically impossible to lose 30 pounds of fat in 30 days. To lose weight, you have to create a calorie deficit, either by lowering your calorie intake or by burning up more calories through increased physical activity. You need a deficit of 3,500 calories to lose 1 pound. To lose 30 pounds, you would need a deficit of 105,000 calories. The average person eating 2,800 calories a day consumes only 84,000 calories in a month. The bottom line is that you could stop eating and still would have to burn an additional 21,000 calories to lose 30 pounds in 30 days. That's about 70 hours of brisk walking. You can see how ridiculous a claim like this is once you do the math.

Finding Out the Truth

The first problem with going *on* a diet is that sooner or later, you'll have to go *off* that diet. You need to look for a lifelong approach to weight management, but how can you tell whether a program has live-with-it-for-life potential? Take this quick quiz from Ann Ruelle, R.D., of Advanced Healthcare, S.C., in Milwaukee and co-author of the TOPS Club guide, *The Choice is Yours.*

1. How does this affect my food choices?

Fads tend to limit our food choices. Look for a plan where anything goes. You can't go through the rest of your life without eating your favorite foods. All foods should be legal.

2. Is this difficult to implement?

Some diets call for hard-to-find foods or hard-to-follow regimens. For example, the Sugar Busters! plan suggests eating alligator, elk, and quail. Can you find these meats in your local grocery store? Losing weight is difficult enough. The easier a program is to follow, the more likely you'll be to stick with it, says Ruelle.

3. Will this program affect my health?

The next thing you should consider is the health benefits of a diet. Can you answer, "Yes, I will be better off than I am today because this plan will benefit my health"?

4. Will it control my weight?

This is actually the last point to ponder, not the first, says Ruelle. Before you can start to think about weight loss in terms of numbers on a scale, you need to decide to change your lifestyle. And that lifestyle change needs to be one that is not just effective but also good for you in the long run.

All the Things You Are: Taking Personal Inventory

W ho are you?

No, don't list your physical attributes, job, and number of kids. Who are you *really*? Until you can answer that question with the kind of soul-searching self-evaluation and honesty it requires, you'll never be permanently successful in your weight loss quest.

"You really have to get acquainted with yourself," says Cheryl Rock, Ph.D., associate professor of family and preventive medicine at the University of California, San Diego. "This personal assessment is the absolute first and most important step in the weight loss process."

Like unfolding a map and trying to decipher which direction is north, we need to know where we are before we can decide where to go. We need to look at our eating patterns, think about the ways we like to have fun, and understand how we react to stress. We need to consider whether our goals are realistic and if we're ready to take the time to achieve them.

So get a pencil and paper and spend some time with someone you may barely know—yourself.

How Much Weight Do I Need to Lose?

This is the first question we should ask when we tackle a weight loss program, says Howard J. Rankin, Ph.D., behavioral psychology advisor for the TOPS club and author of 7 *Steps to Wellness*. "The question should be, 'What level of eating and exercise can I realistically expect to maintain?' The secret to being successful at weight control is to recognize what is possible for you and to set up your program accordingly."

For instance, if you're currently eating an average of 2,500 calories a day and the couch has a permanent imprint of your body, then deciding to suddenly go on a 1,200-calorie-a-day diet and jog 2 miles a day is probably a recipe for failure.

So start small and move up incrementally. And be specific. Instead of declaring, "I'm going to eat healthier and exercise more," make a pact with yourself to eat at least ½ cup of vegetables each day. Or exercise an additional 5 minutes every other day. When you can count these small successes, it's easier to overlook the inevitable backsliding.

WHAT'S YOUR BMI?

Body mass index (BMI) is a more valuable measurement of health risks than your bathroom scale. Higher BMI numbers are associated with greater death rates and risk of diseases, including high cholesterol, high blood pressure, heart disease, stroke, diabetes, and certain cancers.

Here's how to calculate your BMI.

1. Multiply your weight in pounds by 0.45 and then round it to the nearest whole number. For example, 150 pounds × 0.45 = 68. This number represents how much you weigh in kilograms.

2. Multiply your height in inches by 0.025. For example, if you're 5 feet 6 inches tall (66 inches), 66 × 0.025 = 1.65, your height in meters.

3. Square the answer from step 2 (1.65 × 1.65) = 2.72

4. Divide the answer in step 1 by the answer in step 3 (68 ÷ 2.72 = 25) This is your BMI.

A healthy BMI should fall below 25 advises Carol Boushey, Ph.D., assistant professor in the department of foods and nutrition at Purdue University in West Lafayette, Indiana. If you score 25 or more, you should lose enough weight to lower your BMI at least one or two numbers.

And whether you're trying to drop 5 pounds or 50, don't overrate the importance of that goal weight, says Sandra Haber, Ph.D., a New York City psychologist who specializes in women's weight issues. "The idea of judging yourself by a number on the scale is a very important thing *not* to do." she says. "Weight is just one component of who you are, how you appear to others, and how you appear to yourself."

Focusing all your energy on reaching a goal weight and then not getting there—or not getting there fast enough—can feel overwhelming. The result is that you're more likely to give up, says Dr. Rankin. And this is going to take time. For instance, a moderately active woman who eats 1,200 calories a day will probably lose 3 pounds a month.

Am I Doing This for Me?

If you're trying to shed pounds because other people think you should or because a family member has been bugging you about it, you're less likely to succeed than if you're doing it for yourself.

Listen to what you say for clues about your motivation. For example, when you told your best friend about your weight loss plan did you say, "I *should* lose weight" or "I *want* to lose weight?"

"When you hear someone say, 'I should lose weight,' that's usually a bad sign," says Dr. Haber. "*Shoulds* tend to be things that we think in our heads that we may or may not do. I *should* because it's healthy, or I *should* because I'll look better, or because I can't zip my pants anymore. There's a lot of *shoulds* in life, and we don't do most of them."

Saying "want," however, signifies that you're doing this for yourself—and that's an important first step in losing weight.

Is This the Right Time to Make Lifestyle Changes?

Timing is everything when you're charting your weight loss strategy. Are you in the middle of a kitchen remodeling job? Leaving in a couple weeks for vacation? Then it's not the time to start changing your lifestyle habits.

"You want to embark on a weight loss program when the rest of your life is as normal as possible," says Janet R. Laubgross, Ph.D., a clinical psychologist specializing in weight loss in Fairfax, Virginia.

Major changes in your life like a new job, a move to a new residence, a marriage, or a divorce raise stress levels. Pile more changes on top of that, like a new exercise routine, and you're likely to become overwhelmed and quit.

"Weight loss in itself is a stressor," says Dr. Laubgross. It gobbles up precious time in your already overbooked schedule. You may have to shop more frequently for fresh produce, carve 10 minutes from your lunch hour to take a walk, or sit down for a half-hour each week to plan healthy menus.

"When we ask ourselves, 'Is it the right time?' we should also be asking ourselves, 'Is this a time when I'm ready, willing, and able to take the time I need to make permanent lifestyle changes?'" says Dr. Laubgross.

Do You Know Your Favorites?

While it's important to eat low-calorie foods when we're trying to lose weight, it's much more important that we *like* those calories.

Usually, we don't. We go on a diet and eat prescribed foods as if they were medicine—foods that we have no intention of eating after the diet

WOMEN ASK WHY

Why do women like to talk about food more than men?

For a hundred different reasons. Unlike men, women are taught to think about food from a very early age through images we see in magazines and television. Think about your first Easy Bake Oven.

By age 8 or 9, young girls already understand the connection between food and their bodies, and they often begin dieting. So there's an early understanding of food and weight issues and how they are interrelated.

Then there's the role that food plays in our daily lives. We're the caretakers and nurturers, and food is one way for us to show our families that we're taking good care of them. It's also an inescapable element of our daily lives. We keep the grocery list, plan the menus, and trudge out to the grocery store. We stock the pantry and the refrigerator. We remember to take the chicken out of the freezer so there will be something for dinner when we get home. And once the dinner hour rolls around, we're more likely to be doing the cooking. If we have children, we typically decide whether they're going to eat "Super Sweet Sugar Crisp" for breakfast or "Bran Flakes."

Even if we're ordering take-out food from a restaurant, we're in charge of what the family will eat. Because we're constantly involved with it and always thinking about it, somewhere along the way, it's going to come up in our conversations.

Men, on the other hand, don't have a clue. They don't usually care what they're eating, how it got there, or what preparation went into it. When they run out of bologna, they expect it to just magically reappear in the refrigerator. Then when they gain a few pounds, they wonder, "How did I gain this weight?"

Expert consulted
Sandra Haber, Ph.D.
Psychologist
New York City

is over. Then we can't wait to go off the program. So what's the point?

To design a program that includes foods that you like best, rate the foods you eat on a scale of 1 to 10. A 1 is a food that you absolutely hate. A 10 is a food that you absolutely love. "I ask people to design diet programs with foods that are minimally a 6 and optimally a 10," says Dr. Haber. "We're looking for foods that nurture them, that taste good, and that they will continue to eat once they've lost the weight," she says. Now, if their top five foods are things like Cheetos, chocolate cake, and Big Macs, Dr. Haber works with them to identify other, less fattening foods that they also enjoy.

How Much Activity Do You Get?

Chances are, not enough. Only about one in four of us gets the 30 minutes of daily activity that health experts recommend. Lack of activity is one of the main reasons why we gain weight as we get older, says Miriam Nelson, Ph.D., associate chief of the Human Physiology Laboratory at the Jean Mayer USDA Human Nutrition Research Center on Aging at Tufts University in Boston and author of *Strong Women Stay Slim.*

Even if our jobs keep us chained to our desks all day, we have to consciously choose ways to work activity back into our lives, advises Dr. Nelson. We have to get up more, walk more, take the stairs more.

To get her clients moving, Dr. Haber again asks them to pinpoint the pleasure factor of various activities on a scale of 1 to 10. If you ab-

WOMAN TO WOMAN

She Was Eating to Relieve Stress

Carole DeMartino, a 55-year-old laboratory manager from Bloomfield, New Jersey, calls her 120-pound weight loss a midlife miracle. Dieting, she says, has nothing to do with your stomach and everything to do with your brain. Here's her story.

When I was a child, I used to go to sleep praying for a miracle—that I'd wake up and the rest of the world would be fat, too.

I got fat when I was 2 years old, and I stayed fat. I was the kid who had to shop in the chubbette section for a dress. When I was in eighth grade, I went on my first diet. My mother took me to the doctor, and he prescribed amphetamines. Of course I lost weight—I didn't eat or sleep. But as soon as I went off the pills, the weight came back. By the time I got to high school, my nickname was Carole Barrel.

Growing up fat was stressful, and I learned to use food to soothe that stress. On the outside, I was a jolly, flamboyant fat person. But I was miserable on the inside. No one saw me eat. I'd skip my meals all day, and then go home and pig out every night.

Food was my comfort. I became a food addict. Even a gallon of ice cream wasn't enough. My life was one big eating marathon.

solutely hate aerobics class—if it rates a 1—don't bother going. But if you love belly dancing, take a couple of classes. It's not important that aerobics burns more calories. What's important is finding an activity that will stay on your calendar and fit into your lifestyle.

How Supportive Is Your Environment?

"Think about the people in your environment," says Dr. Rankin. Make a list of who is

One day, I decided to weigh myself. I weighed 265 pounds. That shocked me into the recognition that I was killing myself. Because I manage a medical lab, I knew all along that my numbers weren't good. I was 50 years old and had high blood pressure, high blood sugar, and extremely high cholesterol. I realized at that point that I had to do something.

I started out saying, "Let's see what I can do one day at a time." I went on a cabbage soup diet and lost 15 pounds. That was what I needed to get started. I adopted a low-fat, high carbohydrate eating plan and eventually became a vegetarian. In 18 months, I lost 120 pounds.

Instead of eating to cope with stress, I exercised every day. At first, I simply walked around the block. Now, I lift weights twice a week and walk for an hour each day. The outdoors is my gym. I've never felt better. My blood pressure and blood sugar are normal and my cholesterol is down to 180.

Being thin hasn't made stress evaporate from my life, but I've learned to deal with it differently. Some nights, I come home from work so stressed that I'm just crying to eat. I've found ways to break that cycle. I rinse my mouth out with water or brush my teeth. Then I go for a 60-minute walk. All that negative energy dissipates and is replaced by positive energy. Exercise is just plain good for your soul.

supportive and positive and who is sabotaging you. One person could be both. Maybe you and your husband enjoy dinner out three or four nights a week. He may not want you to change your eating habits if it means that he has to change his routine, too. On the other hand, he may help you work in physical activity by asking you to go for a walk after dinner.

Decide how you're going to handle those situations. Overall, you really do need support if you're going to change your lifestyle. Women tend to do better at weight loss when they have some type of support network, so ask for it.

Maybe you can get it from people at home, or your friends or coworkers, or from a group like TOPS, says Dr. Rankin.

Do You Expect to Be a Perfect Dieter?

Let's say you have a party and a friend brings your favorite dessert—apple pie. You can't resist, and you have not one but two pieces. "I really blew it today," you say to yourself. You now have two choices: Get rid of the leftover pie and get back on your program the next morning. Or, you may figure what's the use, and eat the rest of the pie. Usually, we do the latter. Weight loss experts even have a name for it: the I'll-diet-tomorrow effect.

The real problem isn't the extra piece of pie. Everybody is going to overeat at some time, even skinny women. "What really counts is how quickly you get back on your feet," says Dr. Haber.

So don't berate yourself. "Being a harsh, critical taskmaster never does anybody any good," she says. "It doesn't boost you up. It's defeating and negative."

Instead, find a way to deal with the situation in the most positive, optimistic way you can. In the apple pie situation, you can learn from the problem and offer to make the desserts next time.

Can You Remember Everything You Ate Today?

If the answer is no, then you're not paying enough attention to what you're putting in your

WHAT'S YOUR BODY IMAGE?

What do you see when you look in the mirror? Almost everyone has something about their bodies that they don't like. In a survey conducted by *Psychology Today*, 56 percent of women were dissatisfied with their overall appearance. Nearly two-thirds were dissatisfied with their weight.

Did you know that learning to like your body can double your chances of getting slimmer?

Researchers at Stanford University School of Medicine found that people who started a weight loss program feeling happiest with their bodies were more than twice as likely to lose weight as those who were least satisfied with their bodies.

Here's how to get happy with your body *before* you lose weight.

Accept your power. Self-image has a lot to do with what we say to ourselves internally, says Judy Schiller, Ph.D., a clinical social worker and psychoanalyst in San Francisco. Women who like their bodies tend to have an easier time losing weight. If a woman has a poor body image, the real problem is how she feels about herself. To be successful, she has to change the message to herself and say, "I am a good person, and I don't have to lose weight to feel valuable." Either way, she needs to take control of the situation and understand the underlying feelings that are getting in the way of controlling her weight. Then a weight control plan can be successful.

Get moving. To boost your body image and your confidence, get active. But community gyms aren't for everyone, says Michaela Kiernan, Ph.D., a behavioral scientist at Stanford University. You may be more likely to stick with a home-based fitness program such as walking. That way, you don't have to face the stress or embarrassment of a group setting.

We eat in front of the television or while we're standing at the kitchen sink. We wolf down fast food in the car. "The irony is that most people don't really enjoy what they are eating when they eat this way. That's why we eat so much," says Dr. Cross.

To eat less and enjoy it more, you need to find out how much you're eating on a regular basis. The best way to do this is to record everything you eat for the next few days. "When my clients do this, they're amazed at how much they eat," says Dr. Cross.

Do You Eat When You're Bored, Angry, or Stressed?

Emotional overeating protects us from tension and worries, explains Dr. Haber. "As strange as it seems, overeating can be calming; it 'works,' at least in the short run," she says. "And that's why it's a difficult cycle to break."

It's often easier and less upsetting to be angry with ourselves than it is to be tense and angry at an important person in our lives. Often, we transfer our feelings into emotional overeating. The distraction of food, repetitive chewing and swallowing, and obsessive thoughts of food are psychologically safer than confronting our feelings head-on.

The first step in breaking the emotional eating cycle is to understand what feelings you're avoiding, allow yourself to be upset, and then

mouth. Unconscious eating is one of the primary reasons why we gain weight, says Audrey Cross, Ph.D., nutrition professor at the Institute of Human Nutrition at Columbia University in New York City.

choose an alternative behavior to overeating, says Dr. Haber.

Do You Put Everyone Else's Needs First?

Is your pantry stocked with chips and cookies so that the kids have something quick to snack on? Do you serve macaroni and cheese for dinner because it's the only thing everyone will eat without complaint? As women, we tend to put the needs and wants of others before ourselves. Our weight loss efforts are easily defeated when we don't factor our own needs into the equation.

"It's a concept I call healthy selfishness," says Dr. Haber. "For most people in our culture, the word *selfish* has a very negative spin. 'Don't be selfish,' we tell our children. And yet, healthy selfishness is a key concept in self-esteem, in feeling good about yourself, and in making good things happen for yourself."

For example, everyone in the family might absolutely love ice cream. So to be loving and generous, we keep the fridge stocked with fudge ripple. If we don't eat the ice cream, we feel deprived. If we do eat it, we blow our daily calorie count. A better approach might be to buy a lower-calorie treat like frozen yogurt that everyone will enjoy just as much and that we can also eat.

Putting It All Together

The rest of this book is chock-full of tips and advice to help you deal with your answers to these questions. But the underlying theme throughout remains the same: Be kind to yourself.

Weight loss is about nurturing, not depriving. It's about accepting the person you are and making her even better.

PART TWO

The Major Keys of Success

It's the Good Life: See Yourself Thin

In the Japanese martial art of aikido, it's not unusual to see slender, even petite women throwing brawny men twice their size through the air as if they were feathers. How do they do it? In part, through the power of belief and visualization. There is a common saying among the students of this art: "The mind leads the body."

It's true. The mind can lead the body to do amazing things. After downhill champion Picabo Street injured her knee in a 70 mph crash on the Colorado ski slopes in 1996, she had to make some serious changes in her training plans for the 1998 Olympics. She couldn't ski the course in a pre-Olympic race along with her competitors, so instead, she watched videotapes, created an interactive CD-ROM skiing game wherein she coached her players, and visualized skiing the Olympic course again and again and again.

Her mind led her body. Her reward: a gold medal in the 1998 Olympics in Nagano, Japan.

"When we create an image, it helps us focus. It puts our attention on turning the image into reality," explains Lynnette Young Overby, Ph.D., assistant professor of theater at Michigan State University in East Lansing who has studied visualization and used it with her dance students.

If ballet dancers can master complicated routines and Olympic skiers can win the gold and aikidoists can effortlessly toss their opponents, all through the power of visualization, you can certainly use the same techniques to create a happier, more active, and thinner you.

The Mind-Body Partnership

You may think that imagery exists only in your head, but your body knows better. When an athlete imagines sprinting to the finish line, the muscle fibers in her legs start twitching as if she were running an actual race.

The same principle applies to psychological goals, including weight loss. "You're preparing your subconscious mind through the medium of your conscious mind," says Jane Lincoln, who uses guided imagery at the George Washington University Center for Integrative Medicine in Washington, D.C. Once you've prepared yourself with an image of what you want to accomplish, whether that's finishing your first 5-K race or slipping into your sleekest black dress for the annual Christmas party, your body and mind can respond in ways that may turn your hopes into reality.

If you have a good imagination, you'll have no trouble using imagery to help you accomplish your weight loss goals. But if you've never been able to even picture yourself on the beach, feeling the sun on your face and the sound of the waves rolling onto the sand, you might need to get your imagination muscle back into shape.

"Some people naturally form pictures in their minds. Some don't. But imagery is a skill that can be learned," says Kate Hays, Ph.D., a psychologist at the Performing Edge in Toronto, a company that coaches athletes, artists, and business people on improving their performance.

Fortunately, the exercises for this particular "muscle" are fun. To test your visualization ability, try this: Think of a lemon. What does it feel like in your hand? What does the skin look like? Now slice the lemon in half. How does the fruity pulp smell? How does it taste?

After you've finished, think about which sensations seemed most vivid—or most vague. This will give you some idea of which kinds of sensations will come naturally to you in your visualizations and which might need some sharpening, Dr. Hays explains. Maybe you could see the lemon but not feel its pitted skin in your palm. Or maybe you could taste its sour juice but couldn't smell its fresh citrus scent. Learning your sensory strengths and weaknesses is important because of their impact on imagery—and

WOMEN ASK WHY

Why do women lie about their weight while men brag about theirs?

Thin is in." That's what you hear. But it's only true for one sex.

Thin is not in for men—bulk is. And if men can't have muscles, they'll take being a little bigger any way they can get it. For them, being big is about intimidation and strength.

Women, on the other hand, get the message that if you're thin, everything will be okay. Many of our ideals are built around thinness. A woman thinks, "If I were thin, I'd have a better job, I'd have a better love relationship, and I'd feel better about myself." And of course, those things may well come true because when a woman starts losing weight, she starts paying more attention to her appearance. She holds her head higher, and she goes out of her way to meet people. She may attribute her new social success to weight loss, but her change in attitude may have played just as big a part.

Expert consulted
Tracy Sbrocco, Ph.D.
Assistant psychology professor
Uniformed Services University
Bethesda, Maryland

your weight loss success. The more senses you use in your visualizations, the more effective they'll be helping you reach your goals.

Practice, Practice, Practice

"People say, 'Practice makes perfect,'" says Karen D. Cogan, Ph.D., assistant professor of psychology at the University of North Texas Center for Sports Psychology and Performance Excellence in Denton and a former competitive gymnast. "I say, 'Practice makes permanent.'" The more you use imagery, the more effective a part of your weight loss toolbox it will become.

Here are some tips to get you started.

Be sense-ible. When you do imagery, you'll want to draw on all of the traditional five senses: touch, taste, smell, sight, and sound. Then you'll want to add one more: kinesthetic, or how your body feels when it moves.

Lincoln remembers one patient who drew upon her memories of being a dance major in college in her efforts to lose weight. "She imaged who she was in college. She visualized feeling graceful and strong. She pictured the room she used to dance in, right down to the smell of the wood floors. And she told herself, 'I was once that way; I can be that way again.'"

The more senses you involve in your visualizations, whether you're picturing yourself easily refusing second helpings of coleslaw at the company barbecue or enjoying the extra energy that comes with a healthier lifestyle, the more powerful and effective your images will be in making your dreams come true.

Change perspectives. Sport psychologists talk about external imagery, where you see yourself performing an action as though you were watching yourself on TV, and internal imagery, where you imagine the experience through your own eyes. As with your senses, says Dr. Cogan, the more senses you can experience, the more powerful your imagery will be in motivating and supporting your progress toward the life you've always wanted to have.

WOMAN TO WOMAN

Boredom Can Be Beat—And So Can the Munchies That Come with It

For years, Kate Purcell, R.N., of Oklahoma City ate whenever she felt bored. She'd been heavy as a child and was mercilessly teased about it. In the third grade, the other kids dubbed her Fatty Four Eyes—she'd hit 135 pounds and got her first pair of eyeglasses that year. By the time she had her first child at age 22, though, Kate was fed up with being fat. Today, the 49-year-old mother of three weighs 117 pounds and has no time to be bored. Here's her story.

Chocolate. Frozen peanut M&M's. Frozen semisweet chocolate chips. Ice cream. Potato chips. When I was bored, they were all fair game. I would eat and eat and eat, and I never even seemed to notice. It was like I wasn't aware of what I was doing.

I would sit down with a box of six little doughnuts, planning to eat one or two. Then, the next thing I knew, the whole package was gone. When I was bored, food became entertainment, and I would just eat whatever was in the house to keep myself occupied. It was an unconscious reaction. One minute I was in the living room doing nothing, and the next, I was in the kitchen looking for snacks. I didn't realize that I was eating because I was bored.

Like a lot of people who have trouble controlling their weight, I tried going on diets. That started when I was about 13 years old. I tried the grapefruit diet three times, and I even tried a starvation diet, but nothing worked. My weight

Loosen up and breathe. Whatever senses or perspectives you choose to use in your imagery, make sure you're calm and relaxed before you begin to visualize.

To relax quickly and easily, try this breathing exercise, recommended by Simone Ravicz, Ph.D., a licensed clinical psychologist in Pacific Palisades, California, and author of *High on Stress*. Inhale for 5 seconds through your nose. Hold your breath for 20 seconds. Then, exhale for 10 seconds through your nose again, imagwould go down and up and down and up, but it would never just stay down.

I finally got fed up. I was tired of seeing my weight yo-yo, and I didn't like being treated differently from my skinny girlfriends. At age 22, I began to get really conscious about healthy nutrition. And to help me lose weight, I started writing down everything I ate, when I ate it, and how I felt when I ate it. That's when I discovered that I was eating out of boredom.

I started developing a better sense of the real me. I asked myself, "Who am I?" People had called me Fatty Four Eyes, but that wasn't me. I went back to nursing school and got my degree. I learned how to jitterbug with my husband. I connected to the Internet to keep myself out of the kitchen. I also got fashion-conscious and started clothes shopping.

It took me a long time—5 to 6 years—but I managed to lose and keep off 68 pounds, and now I feel great!

The focus of my life is no longer around food. I concentrate instead on my home-based businesses. I'm a national nurse recruiter, and I sell my diet book on the Web.

I still get bored, but I can handle it better now. I keep the tempting foods out of the house. I'll suck on a piece of hard candy. I'll chew gum. I'll grab a Diet Coke. I'll get on the phone and call a friend. I'll fire up my computer and answer some e-mail. I keep lemon drops and cinnamon candies around. And if it gets too bad, I go shopping!

thinks through a race and all its possibilities, from rain to exhaustion and everything in between, you can prepare yourself mentally for dinner with Mom or a difficult meeting with your boss. The result? You'll respond differently and break the cycles that lead to emotion-induced eating.

"It's about changing your lifestyle," says Dr. Ravicz. It's not just about losing weight. "We can create our own reality of what we want our lives to be like."

Perhaps you'd like to dust off your dancing shoes, plant a vegetable garden, or walk after dinner each night. "But I can't," you think. "I haven't danced in years, I know I won't have time to weed, and who will do the dishes?"

Well, just stop. Too often, our negative thinking throws cold water on our ideas before we even have a chance to dream.

To get beyond those automatic thoughts, Dr. Ravicz recommends a visualization that she calls Playing Center Stage. Think of the woman you would like to be. (Feel free to draw on the characteristics of women you admire, whether they're friends, family, public figures, or even a favorite fictional heroine.) What qualities would she have? How would she spend her time? How would she interact with other people? What would her job be? How would she dress? What habits would she have? How would she approach food?

Once you've fully envisioned your ideal self (using all your senses, of course), try actually living a week of your life in her shoes, acting just as you would expect her to act. Freed from the psychological constraints that we all put on our own behavior, you'll try new activities, meet new people, eat new foods, and experience (at least snippets) of a life that you'd only imagined.

ining all the stress melting away. It is important that when you inhale, you breathe from your diaphragm so that your stomach rises, not your chest.

Imagining Your Life

Imagery can help you picture your ideal life and set weight loss goals, but it can also work well for life's everyday challenges, from your workouts to your career. Just as a marathoner

Top TOPS Tips
Her "Dream Album" Helped Her Lose 155 Pounds

Sonia Turner, 43, of Timmins, Ontario, had no trouble imagining herself in a bikini each time she went on a new diet. But the images of a thinner self never seemed to stick, and neither did her diet, until she started her "dream album." Here's how this TOPS member changed her life by harnessing the power of pictures.

"Each time you try to lose weight, you have a mental picture of yourself looking better. That's what motivates you. But if you have a bad day, that picture goes. Your dreams go. I started a dream album to give me visual reminders of what I wanted to accomplish."

Sonia began her dream album with a photograph from her husband's company newsletter. "It was another Christmas when I didn't attend the company dance because I was too self-conscious about my weight," she says. "I weighed close to 300 pounds; nothing looked good on me, and I didn't want to go out." Then the company newsletter arrived, featuring photos of couples dressed to the nines. Sonia decided that she didn't want to miss out on the fun any longer. She cut out the pictures and pasted them into her dream album, adding one line to the accompanying article, forecasting it for the following year: "And also in attendance were Doug and Sonia Turner." "I was going to be at that party," she says.

She filled page after page with similar images of inspiration and motivation. She cut out a photo of a woman wearing jeans, something she hadn't been able to do since she was a teenager. She included magazine stories about women who had lost weight. "I remember one woman named Kathy who had lost 147 pounds and looked fantastic. I'd look at the article and say, 'If Kathy can do it, I can too,'" Sonia says.

She applied the same philosophy toward exercise, pasting photographs of speed walkers and runners into her dream album. Now, the woman who could barely walk around her block runs 5 miles daily and is training for a marathon.

One year and 115 pounds after making her resolution, Sonia went with her husband to his company's holiday dance.

Back to the Future

Now that you've whetted your creative appetite, it's time to harness the power of your imagination to create a detailed, vivid picture of the healthier, active life that you plan to lead.

To create such a picture, pick a day in the future, perhaps a year from today. See yourself waking up, then let your imagination run wild, using the questions below as a starting point. You can, of course, replace these questions with your own to create a more personalized visualization script. You may want to record this script into a tape recorder, leaving pauses after each question to allow yourself time to think about your answers, suggests Dr. Hays.

Morning: How do you start your day? Do you roll out of bed an hour earlier so that you can exercise in the mornings? Do you stretch before you shower? How does it feel to move in your new, leaner body? What does the shower water feel like as it moves over your newfound physique? What outfit do you choose to wear? How does it fit? How does it feel against your skin? What emotions do you feel as you look in the mirror and see the result of your work? What's the expression on your face? What does that high-fiber breakfast taste like?

Mid-morning: How is your day going? What projects are you working on? What did you bring from home for your mid-morning snack? How are you handling the stress of a busy morning? How are people reacting to your directions and ideas?

Noon: How will you use your lunch hour today? What food will you eat? How does it taste to you? How have you made your lunch hour more active? Will you go for a walk after a healthy lunch or perhaps even jog a few miles with a like-minded colleague? What does the outdoors sound like after the hum of your computer? How does it feel to leave work and be active? How does it feel to return to your desk after spending 20 minutes burning calories and stress?

Mid-afternoon: How are you dealing with the mid-afternoon slump? How are you managing the day's workload? How are you handling people's demands?

Early evening: How do you feel after a day's work? Do you go directly home or do you stop at the gym for a quick spin on the stationary bike? What do you do after you arrive home? How do you handle the postwork (and postworkout) munchies? What are your plans for dinner? Will you be dining with your family or hosting friends? What are you (or your spouse) cooking? What aromas can you smell? When you sit down for your meal, what room in your house are you sitting in? What does the table look like? How is the food on your plate arranged? When you take your first bite, how does it taste? What do you talk about at dinner? What (if anything) do you serve for dessert? What are your after-dinner plans?

GUILT-FREE PLEASURE
The Glories of Chocolate

In our heart of hearts, we have always known that chocolate soothes the heart.

Scientists are finally beginning to catch on. In 1996, researchers at the University of California, Davis, found that 1½ ounces of milk chocolate had as many antioxidants as 5 ounces of red wine. These antioxidants, known as phenolics, may protect against heart disease. Chocolate also boasts four times more catechins (another form of antioxidant) than tea and as many polyphenols (yet more antioxidants) as a day's worth of fruits and vegetables. It contains essential minerals such as iron, chromium, copper, and magnesium as well as heart-friendly fatty acids.

As if we needed any more reasons to indulge.

Health benefits aside, nibbling on chocolate doesn't have to wreak havoc with your weight loss plans. In fact, an occasional indulgence might be beneficial. You won't have that feeling of deprivation that often leads to bingeing.

Here are some ways to make chocolate deliver its magic without too many consequences.

Go gourmet. "If you must have chocolate, you want the very best chocolate available in the smallest possible amount," says Laurel J. Branen, R.D., Ph.D., associate professor of food and nutrition at the University of Idaho in Moscow, who admits to a weakness for the tiny Dove Promises. Treat yourself to a truffle at the Godiva counter. You'll feel more satisfied and consume fewer calories. "Imitation chocolate isn't as pleasurable, so you tend to eat lots more of it," Dr. Branen says.

Eat an ounce and stop. It takes about an ounce of chocolate to satisfy a craving and about 30 minutes for your body to realize it, Dr. Branen says.

Go fat-free. In blind taste tests at the University of Missouri in Columbia, people liked the taste of fat-free chocolate ice cream just as much as regular ice cream. Unlike its pale cousin vanilla, chocolate's complex flavor comes from a host of chemical compounds, which make chocolate less vulnerable to "off" tastes in fat-free or low-fat foods.

Night: When you get ready for bed, what pajamas do you choose? As you crawl into bed, how do you feel? What are you thinking as your head hits the pillow and your eyes slowly close?

After you finish this visualization, consider the images that came to mind. Then, grab a pen and paper and start thinking of how you can make this mental picture come true. Hays suggests jotting down the baby steps that you can immediately take toward your goal.

Maybe you want to run a 5-K with your daughter, but the most exercise you get right now is carrying laundry between the kids' bedrooms and the basement. What's the midpoint between yourself right now and the ideal life you pictured just a few minutes ago? After mulling it over, you decide that walking a 5-K represents the midpoint. What can you do to reach that spot between today and the future?

Perhaps you can start by walking for 5 minutes when you have some free time during your day, adding minutes and miles until you reach 3.2 miles (the length of a 5-K). How can you go from that midpoint to your ideal? Maybe you decide to mix walking and running, devising a gradual training program that brings you to the long-hoped-for race date. Through the strength of your own mental images, you can propel your mind and body toward a healthier, slimmer you.

The Way You Look Tonight: Dressing Up Is Slimming Down

Marilyn Monroe was undoubtedly one of the most beautiful women of the 20th century. She was a cinema goddess and a sex symbol. She was also a size 16.

"Women who look good all the time aren't necessarily thin or gorgeous," says Gale Grigg Hazen, a color and image consultant in Saratoga, California, and author of *Fantastic Fit for Every Body*. "But they spend time on themselves, and they pay attention to what looks good on them."

That's hard for most of us. We often feel guilty spending time or money on ourselves, and we may not even know what works best on our fuller figures. We tell ourselves that we'll just wait until we lose weight, and then we'll buy new clothes.

Wrong approach.

Dressing well is just as important as eating healthy. "It's another way of nourishing yourself," says Ruth P. Rubinstein, professor of sociology at the Fashion Institute of Technology in New York City and author of *Dress Codes*.

What's more, the better you look and feel about yourself, says Hazen, the more successful you'll be at losing weight. "If you dress well, you look good immediately. It's not something you have to wait 6 months to lose weight for," says DeeDee, a top plus-size model with the Ford modeling agency in New York City.

So start wearing clothes that flatter your figure *before* you shed a single pound.

Clean Out Your Closet

Before you rush out and buy a new wardrobe, check what's hiding in your closet. Chances are you have some real treasures in there as well as some you'd swear were snuck in by aliens.

Here's how to weed out the good from the bad and the downright ugly.

Invite a friend. Closet cleaning should be fun, says Francine Taylor, stylist of ABC's morning show *The View*. The two of you could open a bottle of wine, put on some dance music, and pretend you're shopping at a fancy boutique. Tell a story about each garment—where you bought it, who you kissed while you were wearing it, what special thing happened to you in it. And don't forget your dresser drawers.

Divide it up. Toss everything into one of three piles—looks great, needs repair, trash—so that everything you put back will look fabulous, Hazen says.

Donate it. Those purple suede bellbottoms? That orange polka-dot rayon dress? The peasant blouse? They're history. Drop them off at a local charity. You'll free up space in your closet and make it easier to find the clothes you do wear, Taylor says. Plus, there's the tax deduction.

If the shoe *doesn't* fit, chuck it. Resist holding on to things from your, ahem, thinner days. The goal is to have a closet full of clothes that fit and flatter your body *right now*, and not to have constant reminders that you're not the weight you want to be. When you get to that weight, you'll have an excuse to go shopping.

Take the 1-year test. Get rid of anything that leaves you thinking, "But it looked good on the mannequin." Don't kid yourself. If you haven't worn it in a year, you're probably never going to wear it again, says Hazen.

Stash it away. If you can't bear to part with certain things, pack them in a box, then date it and store it. If you haven't missed anything in the box after 6 months, haul it off to the Goodwill.

Take it to a tailor. Put aside anything that's missing a button or needs to be altered. If you can't make the repairs yourself, find a good seamstress.

Organize it. At this point, all that's left are outfits that make you look great. So hang like items together—all your pants, shirts, dresses, skirts—arranging them from darkest to lighter colors. "When your clothes are organized, it's easy to see what pieces are missing," Taylor says. Perhaps you don't have a black jacket, or you look great in yellow but don't have a single top in that color. Learning what's in your closet helps you decide what items you need and saves you from buying red shirt number three.

Make a list. Attach pen and paper to the back of your closet door and jot down missing items as they occur to you. It's much easier to remember that you need a brown belt when you're getting dressed and realize that all you have is black.

HOW TO LOSE 5 POUNDS
INSTANTLY FROM YOUR FACE

In a 1999 interview on *60 Minutes II*, Jodie Foster's face looked flawless. And no wonder—her makeup job cost $3,000.

For celebrities and models, wearing makeup is more than smearing foundation over their skin to hide blemishes and brushing mascara on their lashes to make them look longer. It's a way to slim down their cheeks, camouflage a double chin, and brighten their eyes, says Diane Irons, an international image consultant to celebrities and models and author of *9·1·1 Beauty Secrets*.

Maybe you can't afford the fancy makeup artist, but there are tricks you can steal from the best in the business.

Frame your face. Bring attention toward your eyes. Start by sculpting your eyebrows into a flattering frame by plucking stray hairs and creating an arch. If you have light eyebrows, darken them with an eyebrow pencil with gentle, smooth strokes. Then brush your brows upward, dabbing with hair spray on your fingertips or lip balm to keep them in place.

Emphasize your eyes. Make people look into your eyes—instead of at your round cheeks and double chin—by brightening them. Line the lower rim of your eye with a white pencil, then curl your upper lashes. Then apply a light shadow to the inner part of your upper eyelid and a darker, neutral color in a V shape that comes to a point on the outside of your lid. Finally, add two coats of mascara.

Place your powder where it counts. Where you put translucent powder has a lot to do with how thin your face looks. Putting it on the tip of your chin elongates your face. From your brows to the tip of your nose, powder narrows your nose. And sweeping it just below the outer portion of your eyebrow arch brightens your eyes. Use loose powder that either matches or is one shade lighter than your skin tone, Irons suggests. "Our trick to making it last is to spray a little aerosol hair spray on the powder puff before putting it in the powder."

Hide round cheeks. The number one slimming tool in your makeup bag is bronzing powder. Find an inexpensive shade that's one or two shades darker than your foundation and run it just under your cheekbone to slim your cheeks. Line it just below your jaw to hide a double chin. You can also brush it down the sides of your nose to narrow it.

Pout. Draw attention from full cheeks by playing up your lips. Dab petroleum jelly on them and brush with a toothbrush to get rid of chapping and make them puffier. Then, gently line the outside of your lips with a neutral liner. Fill in with color and add a little more petroleum jelly. Your model-like pout should last about 4 hours.

Mark your calendar. Now that your closet is neat and tidy, the key to keeping it that way is to check back every 3 months. It's like cleaning out your refrigerator, only there shouldn't be anything moldy to throw out. Note any new items you need, and check the condition of the things you wear frequently. Collar fraying on your favorite white blouse? Toss it and get a new one.

Now it's time to fill in the holes. Get your credit cards ready and let's shop.

Take the Misery Out of Shopping

Most women love to shop. The problem is that when we're overweight, the thought of trying on clothes under harsh fluorescent lighting in front of cheap, three-way mirrors in overheated dressing rooms is enough to send us screaming for chocolate. Well, there's a way to deal with that problem. If you try on only the clothes that are right for you, you may be surprised at what your reflection shows. "By using a few fashion tricks, you can look up to 20 pounds thinner," says Diane Irons, an international image consultant to celebrities and models and author of *911 Beauty Secrets*. Here are some of the tricks she's talking about.

Bring your best friend. Husbands won't do. They have too much at stake to be totally honest. You need someone who's not afraid to tell you that those pants aren't the most flattering on you, or that sleeveless shirts don't make the most of your shape. Otherwise, you'll wind up with another outfit you'll never wear.

Get comfortable. Wear an outfit that's easy to take on and off, such as a button-up blouse, slip-on shoes, and pull-on pants. And wear the right things *under* your clothes, including panty hose and a well-fitted bra. "They'll have a tremendous effect on the way the clothes fit," Hazen says.

Resist buying on impulse. When you buy something on a whim, there's a good chance that it won't match anything in your closet once you get it home. So make a shopping list before you leave the house so that you have a clear idea of what you're looking for.

WOMEN ASK WHY

Why don't women get the message that many men prefer women with a few extra curves?

The old saying, "You can't be too thin," doesn't hold true with many men. They still prefer their women larger than we think they do. The proof: When men choose from a range of body shapes that they think are attractive, they pick larger silhouettes than women think men prefer.

So why don't women feel like goddesses when they have curves that would make Rita Hayworth swoon? Because that's not today's fashion. The ideal body type seen on television and in magazines is such an unrealistically thin standard that even models and actresses must work unbelievably hard to live up to it.

Because most of us are shorter and heavier than a 5-foot-9-inch supermodel with "perfect" 34-24-34 measurements, we end up feeling bad about our bodies, regardless of how many times our husbands compliment our shapes. If we recognize that we tend to have distorted images of ourselves and stop trying to meet the unrealistic expectations that we (wrongly) think others have of us, then we can more easily work toward self-acceptance.

Expert consulted
Stacey Tantleff Dunn, Ph.D.
Assistant professor of psychology
University of Central Florida
Director of the Laboratory for the Study of
*   Eating, Appearance, and Health*
Orlando

Test the fit. Wearing clothes that fit well is the single most important step to looking good, says Hara Estroff Marano, author of *Style Is Not a Size.* "Clothes that are too tight or too big make you look larger than you really are."

- Shirts or blouses: Reach both arms above your head to see if you have enough room under the arms. Also, make sure that there's no tugging around your bust and that when you put your arms down, the sleeves fall around your wrist bone.

- Jackets and overblouses: They should end at your hips. Most important, the shoulder line should be just at the edge of your shoulders. "Shoulders really have to fit neatly. They can't be sloppy, because the shoulder line creates the dominant line in a garment," Marano says.

- Pants, skirts, and dresses: Bend down as if you're picking something up off the floor. If there's a chair or bench in the dressing room, sit down. You should have enough room to move around freely without feeling as if something might pop or tear, says Irons.

- Waists: To check the fit, slip two fingers in the waistband. Pull ½ inch of fabric out at both hips to make sure that it's not too tight. And before taking off the dress or pants and buying them, check to make sure that the back looks as good as the front.

Take a tote. Bring with you anything you're trying to match. That way, you're not guessing at colors, and you can make sure that the item you're buying works with what you already have. Also, bring shoes to try on with the outfit and a comb or brush to fix your hair between outfits.

Size things up. Be open to trying on several sizes. Are size 16 pants too long? Try a 16 petite. Is size 12 a bit snug? Try a 14. Don't get upset if you have to go up a size, Hazen says. Your size is bound to be different from one clothing line to the next because there's no set standard for sizing among manufacturers. Besides, the size on the tag isn't what matters. "Don't go for the size; go for the fit," she advises.

Ask for help. The sales clerks can be your best ally. If the store doesn't have something in your size, the clerk may know when they'll be getting more, or she can call around to other stores to find it, DeeDee says. They'll call you when it comes in.

Lower your expectations. Clothes are cut for the "average" woman. The problem is that there is no average woman. That's why it's so hard to find clothes off the rack that fit us perfectly. "If you expect that most things won't fit, you won't get frustrated and quit," Hazen says. Instead, you'll be delighted when you find one or two things that do fit well.

Styles to Suit Your Shape

The secret to looking spectacular no matter what your size or shape is to show off your best features, DeeDee says. If you have great legs, wear skirts hemmed above the knee. Gorgeous eyes? Wear something that matches their color close to your face.

VANITY SIZING: WHAT'S GOING ON?

We all know the exhilaration of slipping into a pair of jeans that are a size smaller than what we normally wear. No matter what the scale says, that number on the clothing tag is what we listen to. And it says we're thinner than we thought we were.

If only it were true.

The sobering news is that our clothes are growing with us. A size-12 woman in the 1950s had a 24-inch waist. Today it's 28.

As our bodies grew over the decades, so did our sensitivity about the number on the size tag. So clothing manufacturers learned that if a size-12 woman could fit into a size-10 pair of jeans, she would be more likely to buy them, says Margaret Voelker-Ferrier, chairperson of the fashion design program at the University of Cincinnati. Before we knew it, clothes grew so much that women who normally wore a size 2 were now nearly into negative numbers.

In fact, says Voelker-Ferrier, we've become so obsessed with size that many of us refuse to buy anything bigger than the magic number that we've set for ourselves.

We're paying a price for that smaller number. A roomier size 8 costs more than a "true" size 8, says Gale Grigg Hazen, a color and image consultant in Saratoga, California, and author of *Fantastic Fit for Every Body*.

The most expensive dress that most of us will ever buy is the exception. Yup, don't be surprised if you order your wedding dress 2 sizes larger than you think you wear. Wedding dresses are still cut to the standards of the 1950s, when a 12 was today's size 8, says Hazen.

The best way to avoid letting vanity sizing affect you is to simply stop worrying about what the tag says. "Concentrate on what fits and flatters you, even if that means you're wearing a blouse, skirt, and jacket of all different sizes," Hazen says.

"You don't have to be cookie-cutter pretty to look pretty amazing," Irons says.

If you're not sure what your best features are, ask someone you love and trust. Then use these

REAL-LIFE SCENARIO

Clothes in Her Size Depress Her

Hannah, 38, is a dreamer. Every month, year after year, she buys a half-dozen fashion magazines. She looks at the clothes, lingers over them, imagining what they would feel like against her skin, how the fabric would smell, and what kind of accessories would work with them. And just for a moment, she'll imagine how great she's going to look in them someday. The problem is that someday never seems to come. For now, she has to be satisfied with a closet full of clothes designed for plus-size women, and just the sight of them depresses her. There's something about the very size of those clothes, compared with the ones in the magazines, that makes her feel doomed to be overweight forever. And when she feels that way, she eats to make herself feel better. What can she do?

Hannah is comparing herself with a world that doesn't exist: the world of fashion magazines. Only one-quarter of 1 percent of the female population qualifies to be a fashion model, so Hannah is not looking at a realistic picture of women.

She needs to realize that just because she's never going to look like the models in the magazines doesn't mean that she can't wear sexy and flattering clothes. There are a lot of women who have a closet full of plus-size clothes who feel and look great. Hannah needs to take some lessons on how to feel like a diva instead of feeling dumpy.

She should prominently display a flattering picture of herself that reminds her of a happy time in her life to build her confidence. And instead of focusing on the unrealistic body shapes that she sees in magazines, she should find real role models, like Oprah Winfrey or plus-size model Emme Aaronson.

Then, when she stands in front of a mirror, Hannah should look at what's beautiful about her body instead of focusing on her shortcomings.

Expert consulted
Judith Ann Graham
Owner
Judith Ann Graham, Image Consultant
New York City

fashion-forward tips and our garment-by-garment guide to find a look that you can love.

Create a signature style. Once you find a look that works for you, duplicate it. "I call it developing a uniform," Hazen says. A "uniform" makes picking out something to wear a snap. DeeDee, for example, always wears black pants and dress boots with a V-neck cashmere sweater or a blouse with a shell underneath.

Start with seven. To build a beautiful wardrobe, start with these basic pieces: a white shirt; a grey pants suit; a sweater; a black skirt, jacket, and pants; and black boots or heels. "You can make it through a whole year just by mixing and matching these seven pieces," Taylor says. The sweater should be a color that looks good on you, she adds, and it can be a cardigan, V-neck, or turtleneck—whatever flatters you most.

To add variety to your wardrobe, accessorize with scarves, jewelry, and different types of tops. But stick to items that are classic rather than trendy. "The trendy items will be out of style in a few months, but classics never go out of style," Taylor says.

Find the right fabric. Stay away from those that cling rather than drape, stiff materials that form harsh lines or boxy looks, and bulky clothes that add visual pounds, Marano says. Stick with fabrics that create smooth, clean lines, like wool and silk crepes, Lycra, cotton and rayon blends, and gabardine. They may cost a little more, but they're a better investment in the long run.

With no angles or edges, this fabric flows from the hand like a waterfall. The more a fabric drapes, the narrower the fall.

This fabric hangs easily without gapping or bunching.

A fabric that drapes will fit the shape of your hand. You should feel no resistance, as this fabric will not take up much space.

Pick small prints. Sometime in the distant past, we got the idea that we should never wear prints. "You *can* wear prints—just choose smaller patterns and make sure that the print is on the slimmest part of your body," Irons says. So if you're wider at your hips than your chest, wear a printed top with a solid skirt.

Fix the fit. Sleeves that are too long can easily be shortened, and roomy pants can be hemmed or taken it. These alterations make a world of difference, Hazen says. You instantly go from looking sloppy to looking put together.

Stick with steam. Wrinkles ruin the drape of a garment. To keep clothes wrinkle-free, hang them up as soon as you take them off. Still wrinkled? Use a hand steamer instead of an iron. It's quicker, and the moisture prevents static cling, says Julie Alderfer, head of wardrobe for the television program *The View*. Or, hang your clothes in the bathroom when you shower and let the steam do its work.

Blouses and Tops

Full-busted or flat as Kansas, what you wear on top can serve to enhance your look. Here's how.

Know your necklines. V-neck and surplice necklines are especially slimming, Marano says,

Surplice neckline

because they create vertical and diagonal lines that make you look longer and thinner through the torso.

Slim with sleeves. Tapered sleeves make your arms look longer and more slender, Marano says. Sleeves with broad cuffs, however, shorten the line of the arm and add weight to your hips when your arms are at your sides.

Reshape your shoulders. Give rounded shoulders a more flattering shape by choosing set-in sleeves rather than drop sleeves, Marano says. Set-in sleeves attach at the shoulder, whereas drop sleeves start below the shoulder. Shoulder pads can also reshape shoulders and make your upper body look more proportionate with your hips. But bigger is not better. "They only add bulk," says Irons. Replace large pads with small round ones that conform to your shoulders, she suggests. Look for them at sewing and fabric stores.

Pass on pockets. If you're full-figured, avoid wearing shirts or blouses with breast pockets. They'll only make you look bigger, Irons says. By the same token, you can maximize a small bosom with breast pockets and large shirt buttons.

To tuck or not to tuck. If you have a defined waist, tucking in your shirt creates a flattering hourglass shape, DeeDee says. But avoid this trick if you're larger around the middle.

Grow with a tank. If you're short-waisted, wearing a silk, satin, or knit tank top under a jacket adds length to your neck and torso, Taylor says.

Jackets

A good-quality jacket is a key staple in every woman's wardrobe. "It takes you everywhere," Irons says. You can wear it with a skirt, pants, or even over a dress. And unlike other articles of clothing, jackets can be tailored many times, which is handy when you're losing weight. Here are Irons' suggestions for finding the right jacket for your wardrobe.

Pick the perfect cut. If you're large-busted, avoid double-breasted jackets and breast pockets. They make full-figured women appear larger than they are. Instead, go with a tuxedo-cut jacket, which makes you look taller and thinner.

Tuxedo-cut jacket

Seek out seams. Look for a jacket that has a line of buttons or vertical seams down the front. These elements visually lengthen your torso and have a slimming effect.

Trim with a nip and a tuck. Jackets with a gently nipped-in waist trim the middle of your body and are very stylish.

Consider a knit. A knit jacket won't wrinkle and can be very slimming if it skims the body rather than clings to it.

Dressing Up

There's much to consider when choosing skirts and dresses. What are your hips like? Your stomach? Your waist? Your answers will determine what you buy.

Forgo flared. A-line and flared silhouettes like the one pictured here add width to your hips. Instead, choose skirts and dresses that are tapered slightly in from the hips. "A tapered skirt really flatters your legs and gives your body a very long, narrow look," Marano says.

A-line skirt

GUILT-FREE PLEASURE

Rent a Fabulous Gown

You're eating at an elegant restaurant, candlelight setting your skin aglow, the perfume of roses filling the air, and your husband, dashing in a black tuxedo, by your side. And you—you're looking gorgeous in an ankle-length, deep-blue velvet dress with a heart-shaped top and sexy spaghetti straps.

The best part—you didn't spend hundreds of dollars on a dress that you might never wear again. For about half the cost of buying a gown, you rented this one for a magical 24 hours.

And you don't have to be a size 6 to enjoy this scene. In fact, the better you look in your size right now, the more confidence you'll have in losing weight. Although rental boutiques may not be easy to find, check bridal stores and evening-wear departments for leads. Then flirt, dance, and avoid cream sauces (if you stain the dress, you'll have to pay for them to have it cleaned).

Here's how to look great in a gown if you have a few pounds to hide.

Aim for A-line. Avoid feeling confined in a straight dress and go for the roomier A-line cuts in gown lengths. They'll flatter your figure and give you more freedom below your waist. Avoid A-line skirts, however; they have the opposite effect.

Show your shoulders. Choose spaghetti straps or tank-style tops with a scoop neck for a sexy look. If you're uncomfortable showing a lot of skin, wear a shawl or a bolero jacket.

Shoot for simplicity. If you don't want to look overdressed, avoid sequins and flashy material. For a simple and elegant look, choose satin, velvet, or polyester blends. For a more formal look, wear gloves and a scarf.

Stay comfy. Rent a stretch velvet dress. The material stretches with you and isn't confining, leaving more room for dancing.

Show some leg. If you have great legs, draw attention to them by wearing skirts and dresses hemmed above the knee. If you're short, stick with longer skirts to make you look taller and thinner.

Slim with a slit. A front slit creates a long vertical line that is very slimming, Irons says.

Wrap it up. Wrap skirts are another slimming choice because they form a long vertical line where the two skirt panels overlap, Marano says.

Pants

Ever put on a pair of pants that fit, yet didn't do you justice? Whether you're looking for jeans or dress pants, these tips will help you pick a pair that flatters your figure.

Play it straight. Bellbottoms may have made their way back into style, but we don't have to be enablers of bad fashion. Stick with straight-leg pants, Irons says, for a slimming line.

Get hip. If you're trying to minimize your hips, pick pants without hip pockets, Taylor says.

Pass on pleats. They draw attention to your tummy. Enough said.

Know whether to buckle up. If you have a defined waist, wearing a belt will accentuate the positive, Taylor says, but belts are usually unflattering for women with larger waists.

Show Your True Colors

Color is the pizzazz that makes an ordinary outfit extraordinary. And while some colors are slimming, others add pounds. Here's how to use the colors in your wardrobe to enhance your figure.

Top it off. Wear bright colors on top and dark colors on the bottom to bring people's attention upward. "If you wear a turquoise shirt with black pants, for example, their eyes will be drawn to your face," Taylor says.

Wear just one. Wearing the same color from your shoulders to your shoes—called monochromatic dressing—streamlines your body by creating one long vertical line.

Match it up. Match your pantyhose to your shoes. It provides that same slimming line of color, Irons says.

Begin with basics. Start with neutral clas-

sics in black, gray, navy, brown, and khaki, then accessorize with color. To add a splash of color, wear a bright top under a jacket, tie a colorful scarf around your neck, or pick an eye-catching purse. "I wear a lot of black, so I get pocketbooks in wacky colors," Marano adds. "It's a modern look and an inexpensive way to update your wardrobe."

Add the Finishing Touches

It's the last thing we do before we run out the door: Throw on some earrings, maybe a necklace, and grab our purse. But these shouldn't be last-minute decisions. "Looking your best is all in the details," Hazen says. Here's how to accessorize your slimming wardrobe with style.

Scarf it up. Knot a long scarf at midchest to trim and elongate your torso. "Go for colorful scarves, because next to your face is a great place to put color," Marano says.

Slenderize with buttons. A vertical line of buttons down the front of a blouse, jacket, or dress is very slimming. "Try replacing the standard buttons with gold or silver ones to really enhance the look of a solid-color suit," Marano says.

Forget about flats. Flat shoes really do nothing for you, Irons says. Heels, however, provide an elegant look that lengthens your legs. Stick with a chunky heel rather than a stiletto for added stability.

Size it right. Larger women can carry off larger accessories, like chunky earrings or bracelets. But use some restraint. "You want your jewelry to be noticeable, but that doesn't mean it should be monstrously large," Marano says.

Go long. When wearing a necklace, choose a long pendant to lengthen and slim your torso, Irons says.

Keep it simple. Whether it's a pin on your

lapel or a bangle bracelet, it's better to wear one piece of eye-catching jewelry than several smaller pieces. "A simple, unencumbered look is very modern," Marano says.

Pick a petite purse. Full-figured women should stick with handbags that are no larger than 10 by 13 inches, Irons says. Anything bigger just adds girth.

Change Your Look with Lingerie

From bras to body slimmers, what you wear under your clothes has a dramatic effect on your appearance. "The right lingerie can really slim and tone you in all the right places," Irons says. "It gives your body a whole new look before you even begin trying to lose weight."

Check the fit. Your bra is one of the most important things you put on. Its fit determines the drape of your sweater or blouse. If you're like most women, you're still trying to squeeze into that 34B you wore when you were 20. In fact, 8 out of 10 women are wearing the wrong size bra, Irons says.

If you haven't been professionally fitted in the past 3 years or so, it's time to get rechecked. You can get fitted at most department stores free of charge.

Banish bulges. Lycra-laced body slimmers and shapers streamline your body and eliminate bulges, Irons says.

Trim your tummy. Control-top panty hose and tummy-toning panties instantly flatten a full waist.

Before
- Drop-shoulder seams
- Breast pocket
- Boxy sleeves
- Wide belt
- Large cuffs
- Busy pattern
- Flared
- Length too long
- Light-colored tights
- Dark-colored flats

After
- V-neck
- Set-in shoulder seams
- Tapered waistline
- Tapered sleeves
- Vertical line of buttons
- Vertical seams
- Flattering length
- Tapered hem
- Dark tights that match shoes
- Chunky heels

Toss unflattering clothes and you can look spectacular—before you lose weight.

Find the Right 'Do for You

We tend to spend more time blow-drying, curling, spritzing, and styling than we do getting dressed. So choose a hair style that flatters your features.

Love your length. A shoulder-length cut flatters a fuller face, says Kim Lépine, hair stylist and owner of salon Lépine in New York City. Put the height on your crown and sides and taper your hair in toward your face at the neck and jaw. If you have long hair, up 'dos that sweep your hair away from your face make your neck look longer, enhancing the perception of thinness. If you have a double chin, draw attention from it with a longer cut that leaves your hair on the nape of your neck, Lépine says.

Say it with style. Go for a look with simple, blunt lines. If you have bangs or a bob, make sure the lines are definite. "When there are too many bangs, too many layers at the wrong places, it doesn't look sophisticated enough," Lépine says. But simple doesn't mean boring. You can add drama with layers or by using Velcro rollers. Just stay away from flips and curls that make your hair look like it's moving in 15 different directions, she says.

Capitalize on color. Be dramatic. If your blond is drab, add highlights to lighten up your face, Lépine says. If you're a brunette, add dimension by highlighting in amber or light brown with a reddish tinge. If your hair is red, add auburn-red highlights, but avoid pink-red or orange-red, advises Lépine.

And remember, once you've found that flattering hairstyle or stunning outfit, wear them with pride. "Two of the most important fashion accessories are posture and a positive attitude," Marano says. "When you look confident, you'll look good in anything you wear."

Feelings: Emotional Eating

For Jan McBarron, M.D., brown sugar was the last straw—or, rather, spoon. As she stood in her kitchen one midnight scooping the sweet stuff out of the box with a tablespoon, she thought: "I can't *believe* I'm doing this." Miserable and 70 pounds overweight, the premed student put down the spoon.

"I was very unhappy, and my weight reflected it," says Dr. McBarron, now director of Georgia Bariatrics, a medical center for overweight people in Columbus, Georgia. A nurse at the time, she was so dissatisfied with her career that she had turned to food for solace.

Yet as her weight rose, her self-esteem plummeted, sending her into a spiral of increasing job frustration followed by more overeating followed by more weight gain . . . until the midnight turning point.

"Like most overweight people, I was trying to feed emotions," she says. Now 70 pounds lighter, Dr. McBarron speaks from experience when she tells her patients that the excess weight often isn't the problem; the hidden emotions are.

Eating Instead of Feeling

For some, it's alcohol or drugs; others escape into work or exercise to avoid feelings that they can't handle. For overweight women, the "drug" of choice is food.

"People who use food to 'numb out' are usually eating to manage negative feelings," says Marlene Schwartz, Ph.D., codirector of the Center for Eating and Weight Disorders at Yale University.

We may feel lonely, angry, or frustrated. Perhaps we're undergoing a major life change—children leaving home, divorce, a career switch. "That's when women are likely to overeat as a way of comforting themselves," says Dr. Schwartz.

This isn't necessarily bad. "To some degree, we all use food for comfort, both physically and psychologically," says Ronni M. Kahn, Ph.D., a psychologist with the Eating Disorders Program of the Richard Young Center in Omaha, Nebraska. Think about comforting yourself with a cup of hot chocolate on a cold winter's day, or the pint of Häagen-Dazs that got you through that breakup with your college boyfriend.

"That's okay," says Dr. Kahn, "unless you reach the point where every hurt, every anger, every everything calls for food. When eating is the only way you can cope, that's a danger signal."

This behavior is frequently found in women with binge-eating disorder, characterized by eating enormous amounts of food within a very short time period. A classic binge might include an entire pizza, a liter of soda, and a gallon of ice cream within an hour.

Asked how they feel after binges, women often answer: "I don't know. I didn't feel anything. I didn't even taste the food," says Dr. Schwartz. "It's as though the extreme overeating is used to escape the awareness of whatever feelings they were having."

"Most women who overeat don't even see the connection between what they're feeling and running to the refrigerator," says Cynthia G. Last, Ph.D., author of *The Five Reasons Why We Overeat*.

"Being overweight in America now is a problem from the chin up, not the chin down," says Dr. McBarron.

Protecting Ourselves with Fat

Maybe you can never be too thin or too rich, but for some women, you can never be too fat. For them, fat serves as a kind of shield against the stresses and disappointments of life.

REAL-LIFE SCENARIO
She Uses Food to Boost Her Mood

Alexis, a 45-year-old homemaker, has lots of time on her hands. Too much time. She gave up a promising career in the airline industry years ago to stay home and raise her only child, Megan, while her husband traveled the country selling copy machines. She and Megan enjoyed a close relationship during those years, remaining the best of friends even through the stress of adolescence. Then everything changed. Megan graduated from a local college and immediately joined the Peace Corps, leaving Alexis alone in a big empty house. That big house had a big refrigerator, and in no time, Alexis made it her new best friend. Whenever she felt down or lonely, she always found something in it to make her feel better. Funny how quickly a plate of cold pasta could make her worries seem so unimportant. Now she has another problem. She has gained weight, she feels heavy, and her clothes don't fit. And she's beginning to feel so depressed that even food isn't helping anymore. What should she do?

Alexis is in what we call role transition: from being a full-time mother to whatever her next stage will be. The problem is that with her child gone, Alexis doesn't have a role to give her a sense of self-identity and self-esteem.

The most effective psychological treatment would involve two steps. First, Alexis needs to evaluate her old role as Megan's mother and best friend and consider what that role meant to her. What were the good things about it—and the bad? Looking at the negatives as well as the positives will help her avoid idealizing that role. It's important that she express how she feels about the change.

"If I'm fat and you don't like me, I can think it's because you're prejudiced against fat people," says Dr. McBarron. "If I lose weight and you still don't like me, then I can't blame it on my fat. So fat can be protective, mentally as well as physically."

That protection can also convey a certain image, says Laurie L. Friedman, Ph.D., deputy

Then, Alexis should find something to get excited about. Now that she has time and energy to focus on something besides being a mother, she needs to identify what that something might be. Returning to the workforce? Volunteering? Joining community programs that have personal meaning for her? The important thing is to stop the downward spiral that she has begun.

The danger of overeating as a way of coping is that the social stigma of being overweight makes it even harder to break out and enter new social situations. Alexis' isolation is a big factor in her depression. There are also questions about what's going on with her marriage. It seems as though her husband is largely absent, and Alexis' need for closeness was met by her daughter. Sometimes when a child leaves home, the parents have to look more closely at their marriage. Is Alexis happy? Does she need to make changes in her relationship with her husband?

Another issue is physical change. At her age, Alexis' metabolism is starting to slow down, so she's apt to gain weight quickly if she doesn't increase her exercise. An ideal solution would be a combination of social and physical activity, like going to a gym, joining a hiking club, or gardening with other women—anything she enjoys.

Expert consulted
Marlene Schwartz, Ph.D.
Codirector
Center for Eating and Weight Disorders
Yale University

director of Johns Hopkins Weight Management Center in Baltimore. "Some women feel that their size commands a certain kind of respect, or that it can be intimidating," she says. Without the extra weight, the women think they don't have that extra impact.

Women, especially those who have been overweight for long periods, may also use body size to avoid sexual involvement. "Women may get more attention from men if they lose weight, and for some, that attention is unwanted. It can be a bit scary," says Dr. Friedman.

Women have to realize that their fat serves a psychological purpose, says Dr. Last. Until they do, they'll never be able to control their eating. And if they do manage to lose weight by focusing on external factors like "bad" food or poor eating habits, she says, this lack of awareness practically ensures that the pounds will return.

"It isn't so much what you eat that's important," Dr. Last says, "but what's really leading to overeating: emotions."

Understanding Your Emotional Triggers

Key to gaining control over your weight is first understanding what triggers your overeating.

Here are some tips to get you started.

Do the write thing. Keep paper and pen next to the refrigerator. "Every time you find yourself there apart from mealtimes, before you eat, think about what's going on and write it down," says Dr. Last. "Did you just argue with your husband? Are the kids screaming?" Eventually, you'll see a pattern. For example: "Every time I'm tense about the kids, I eat."

Make the refrigerator ring. Put a bell on the refrigerator door. It acts like an alarm clock for women who eat in the middle of the night or forage in the fridge unthinkingly.

WHY CAN'T WE LIVE ON LOVE ALONE?

Popular songs, movies, and literature glorify the idea of love as an appetite suppressant. Lovers pining for each other, unable to eat or sleep. Could it be the answer to weight loss?

Maybe. For a little while.

For women who have been focused on weight and food, the dizzying first phase of new romance may offer a temporary solution to overeating, says Susan Olson, Ph.D., a clinical psychologist and weight management specialist in Seattle. But like the phase itself, the effect on hunger is short-lived.

"In a sense, falling in love can help a woman who is an emotional eater," Dr. Olson says. "It's a distraction." Like a child engrossed in play who resists coming in for dinner, a woman in the very first throes of love may be so absorbed with the relationship that food takes a back seat.

The excitement of that first phase of love is like riding a roller-coaster. "Anticipation is a big appetite reducer," says Dr. Olson. If you're feeling butterflies in your stomach and can't think of much except Mr. Wonderful, you may, in fact, be too excited to eat within your normal pattern.

Also, the sexual appetite of new love can overpower our physical appetite for food—but not for long. "As the relationship gets a little more comfortable, even though it's very exciting, the sensuality of food can, in fact, be part of the thrill of a new partner," Dr. Olson says.

"All of the senses are heightened: Everything looks beautiful, you notice flowers, rain is wonderful, and sharing and enjoying food is part of that sensate experience."

Take time out. When stress, boredom, or the blues propel you toward that pint of rum raisin, give yourself time to take control. Cravings often pass within a short time, so set a cooking timer for 10 to 20 minutes and then decide if you still want to eat, says Amy Joye Lund, R.D., nutrition specialist at the University of South Carolina's Weight Management Center in Charleston.

Outplan your appetite. For many women, overeating comes at the end of the workday, when they're home alone in front of the TV. So don't go there, says Lund. "Plan distractions for the times when you overeat," she says. Take a walk or a shower, clean out a closet—any nonfood activity that breaks the emotional eating routine. Plan to eat all your meals at the kitchen table to remove the association between watching television and eating, Lund suggests.

Unlock your food prison. Allow yourself the occasional treat to avoid feelings of deprivation, says Dr. Schwartz. At her Yale weight center, clients who are going to a wedding, for example, are encouraged to have a piece of cake; it prevents overeating later.

Cut yourself some slack. Emotional eaters often have an all-or-nothing approach to a weight loss plan, says Lund. So if they eat a single cookie, they may think, "Well, I blew the day already, I might as well keep going." Keep it in perspective. "Look at that one instance in the context of the rest of the day or the rest of the week and realize how well you actually did. You might not have been perfect, but you weren't a total failure."

Stop feeling like a failure. Feeling like a failure when we eat unhealthily is part of a common, downward spiral in emotional eaters,

Lund says. "A woman might have a burger and fries for lunch and come home feeling guilty for not having done the 'right thing.' Then she feels like she has lost control, so she grabs the Oreos, inhales a dozen or so, and feels even worse. A woman in this situation needs to remind herself that no one is perfect."

"Setting a specific goal related to the behavior that is upsetting her can help," she says. "The goal should be reasonable, without the expectation of perfection. For example, if she has been eating burgers and fries almost every day, she should set a goal to limit burgers and fries to two times a week. Once she meets the goal or sees improvement, she may feel less like a failure."

To Change Eating Habits, Change Emotions

The key, then, is changing our emotional reactions to food, says Fugen Neziroglu, Ph.D., senior clinical director of the Bio-Behavioral Institute in Great Neck, New York.

Dr. Neziroglu uses cognitive therapy, which involves the patient and therapist in an active, goal-oriented approach to solving a specific problem, to help women identify erroneous thoughts or beliefs that may trigger undesirable eating.

So if your boss yells at you and

Top TOPS Tip
She Lost Weight by Following Her Own Rules

It is when she's happy—not feeling stressed or bored—that Marlene Pixley, 56, encounters her eating pitfalls. For more than 23 years, this 5-foot-3-inch homemaker, who coordinates 48 TOPS chapters in Alberta, Canada, has remained at 120 pounds. This is down from her previous weight of 152 pounds. Here's her secret to handling "head hunger."

"I've discovered that when life is good and I'm feeling happy, that's when I do my emotional eating. I went through a divorce 13 years ago and lost weight. When someone in my life dies, I lose weight. So, it's when things are on an even keel that I have to be careful. To do that, I make rules for myself.

"I used to be an evening TV snacker. There was always a bowl of jelly beans next to my chair, or soft cookies, or some cake. So my rule is, no food within easy reach while I watch TV because it gets absorbed by osmosis. I don't even get satisfaction from it because I'm not paying attention.

"Another rule is not eating in my car. Before I started paying attention to what I eat, I'd buy doughnuts and eat half of them—or more—on the way home. It's not that I'm hungry when I see the doughnuts; I simply want them. So now, I usually don't buy them at all. I make sure not to deprive myself, though.

"In social situations or in a restaurant, I'll have the pie or cake (or doughnuts). I know myself well enough to determine what rules I need, so I control my emotions ahead of time by making a conscious decision not to do this or that.

"My rules are mine. I give myself the flexibility to change them when I want to so that I don't feel like I've defeated myself if I break them. They help me set the stage for success."

TYPECAST YOUR EATING TROUBLE

Overeaters who fuel up because of feelings fall into five types, says Cynthia G. Last, Ph.D., author of *The Five Reasons Why We Overeat*. Identify your type (most of us are combinations), and you're halfway to victory.

Impulse eater. You eat while standing up, talking on the phone, or watching TV, but you don't pay attention to how much you're eating.

Type fix: Eat at specific times and places. Don't do anything else while you're eating.

Hedonist. You treat food as pleasure or entertainment, but you gravitate toward high-fat, high-sugar foods. Taste is everything.

Type fix: Turn to alternatives. Get taste appeal from low-fat, low-cal choices like chocolate frozen ice pops instead of high-calorie options like chocolate mousse.

Stress reducer. You use food to relax when you're anxious or tense, but pressure or worry drives you to calorie-dense munchies like candy and potato chips.

Type fix: Defuse your mood with deep breathing, yoga, or exercise (not the chewing and swallowing kind).

Avoider. You use food as a buffer against an unpleasant situation or childhood trauma.

Type fix: Identify your real problems (unhealthy relationship? abusive boss or husband?) and develop problem-solving and assertiveness skills to handle them.

Energizer. You habitually turn to food for a mood lift, resulting in weight gain. Your self-esteem drops and the cycle begins again.

Type fix: Fight a negative mindset with positive thoughts. Browse the "Self-Help" section in bookstores on ways to pulverize pessimism.

you head for the vending machine, what's really going on?

Maybe you feel rejected, says Dr. Neziroglu. "You might say to yourself, 'I'm worthless; everyone is more competent than me' and turn to food to avoid the feeling. That's the way you interpret the situation."

Instead, first try to understand your target trigger. Before you put any money in that vending machine, stop and ask yourself: What just happened? What messages am I sending myself about the situation? What am I feeling?

Then challenge yourself. What thought or belief are you holding on to that may be false? Are you really incompetent, or is the boss just making you feel that way? Does the boss yell only at you, or does she yell at most of the staff? List all the areas in which you feel you are incompetent and all the people your boss yells at, then replay the scene over again in your mind, suggests Dr. Neziroglu. Now how do you feel?

By making the connection between emotions and food, says Dr. Neziroglu, we can "learn to gain control over the food rather than letting our addiction to food control us."

You Can't Take That Away from Me: Eating Well to Lose

We are a generation of women on the go. From the minute our eyes open in the morning to the moment our heads sink gratefully onto the pillow at night, we are racing against time. Between commuting and chauffeuring our kids, we spend 64 minutes a day in the car. At noon, we do everything *but* stop for lunch, squeezing in the dry cleaner, bank, and post office during our average 36-minute lunch "hour."

After work, we hit the grocery store—one of our least favorite errands—sprinting through like a track star, grabbing for milk, bread, and something—*anything*—for dinner. Twenty-four minutes later, we're back in the minivan, wondering why we didn't just order pizza.

The result of our hurry-up lifestyle? Our rapidly expanding waistlines.

"We have worked very hard, practically since we were teenagers," says Irene O'Shaughnessy, M.D., associate professor of medicine at the Medical College of Wisconsin in Milwaukee. "We went to college. We shot for the sky professionally. Now we have families. Understandably, we've started looking for shortcuts, and often these shortcuts involve food."

Breakfast is a cup of coffee. We wolf down lunch at our desks. By the time dinner rolls around, we're famished and exhausted. No wonder we often choose the path of least resistance: fast food, Chinese takeout, or "home meal replacements" from the supermarket.

What we save in time, we gain in weight. Not only do we end up eating too much fat, sodium, and sugar but we also deprive our bodies of the fiber, lean protein, fruits, and vegetables that they need to thrive and stay slim.

But eating a healthy diet doesn't require a Martha Stewart in the kitchen. "No one is saying that women need to start baking bread from scratch again," says Dr. O'Shaughnessy.

Nor does it mean a deprivation diet, dining on celery sticks, cottage cheese, and diet soda until we reach our goal weight. We simply need to make healthy eating a priority in our lives so we can enjoy satisfying meals that include not only food that's good for us, but food that's just plain good.

WOMEN ASK WHY

Why do most diet programs say you must drink eight glasses of water daily?

Because we need to stay well-hydrated. Our bodies are composed primarily of water, and we want to make sure that we constantly flush out the old fluids and refresh ourselves with plenty of new ones.

As a whole, we live in a dehydrated society. We survive on caffeinated products such as coffee, tea, and cola, which make us urinate more often. We drink alcohol, which dries us out. We travel frequently, and the recirculated air involved in air travel can be really dehydrating. Drinking eight glasses of water is just giving you back the minimum that your body needs.

All these dehydrating habits have consequences for our health. When you don't drink enough water, you tend to be thirsty all the time. You may feel tired. Keeping yourself well-hydrated can change that. For example, if you drink a lot of water while traveling by airplane, you'll arrive feeling less jet-lagged. You'll feel more alert and energized. Your skin will look better. And during the cold and flu season, drinking lots of water can minimize your chances of getting sick because it keeps mucous membranes in your nose and throat well-hydrated and better able to resist a virus attack.

Drinking at least eight glasses of water a day is not a weight loss recommendation; it's a health recommendation. If you're well-hydrated, you'll feel better. And if you feel better, you're more apt to be in control of other things—like your weight.

Expert consulted
Franca Alphin, R.D.
Administrative director
Diet and Fitness Center
Duke University
Durham, North Carolina

Never Feel Hungry Again

After starving ourselves on diet after diet, we're ready to take Scarlett O'Hara's desperate vow as our own: "As God is my witness, I'll never be hungry again."

We don't have to be hungry. Losing weight safely and permanently doesn't require starvation diets, grapefruit diets, cabbage soup diets, bacon-and-egg diets, or any other type of "diet." In fact, weight loss experts hate the idea of diets because going on a diet implies that one day we'll go off our diet and return to the same eating habits that contributed to our weight problem in the first place.

"I don't want women to feel hungry. I want them to eat when they feel hungry," says Gail Curtis, director of the weight management program at Wake Forest University Baptist Medical Center in Winston-Salem, North Carolina.

So think long term—changing your lifestyle and eating patterns so you can keep the weight off forever. "You won't have rapid weight loss by eating right and exercising—maybe just a pound a week—but you'll develop habits that are permanent," say Katherine Chauncey, R.D., Ph.D., assistant professor at Texas Tech University Health Sciences Center in Lubbock.

And if you lose weight safely and slowly through better food choices, you shouldn't get those ravenous I-have-to-eat-everything-in-the-cookie-cupboard feelings. Here's how to start.

Make friends with fiber. Get 25 to 35 grams a day, and you'll find that the pounds come off easier and stay off. In one study, people who ate at least 21 grams of fiber a day gained 8 pounds less over a 10-year period than those who ate less than 12 grams. Not only does fiber fill you up on less but it stays with you longer. And numerous studies suggest that it also reduces your risk of heart disease, cancer, and diabetes. Good sources include legumes, fruits, vegetables, and whole grain pastas, cereals, and breads.

Lunch with protein. If pasta salad with a roll represents your typical lunch, add some lean meats or legumes. Research suggests that a high-protein lunch is more filling than a high-carbohydrate one and may also help you eat less at dinner. Add lean turkey breast to your bagel, sprinkle chickpeas on your salad, or toss a carton of low-fat yogurt in your brown bag.

Don't forget fats. This is a tricky one, because eating too much fat is one reason why we're heavy. But women tend to focus on fat and fat alone, ignoring calories, portion size, and exercise in favor of counting fat grams. The result? Frustration.

"I've rarely found a woman who could lose weight successfully by just watching fat grams," says Dr. Chauncey. "Men could make it work, but women rarely could." Men need more calories to begin with, she says, so when they start reducing fat, they really reduce their calories, thus creating a calorie deficit. Women, on the other hand, need fewer calories to begin with, and when they start replacing regular foods with fat-free counterparts, they're not really reducing overall calories that much.

We need a certain amount of fat in our diets. Fat influences the taste and texture of foods and affects how full we feel. Plus, not all fats are "bad." You want to limit the saturated fats, which are found mainly in red meat and other animal products like butter and whole milk. They're the culprit when it comes to artery-

WOMEN ASK WHY

Why do I weigh less in the morning when all I've done for the past 8 hours is sleep?

It's the result of your body's nightly re-balancing act. During the day, you're drinking. You're eating. And your body is slowly but surely metabolizing those calories. As it does this, you're retaining water because water is required to store fat and carbohydrates in the human body. At nighttime, your body settles into a level of homeostasis, or balance, and your kidneys are able to filter out any unnecessary fluids. This allows you to reach probably your lowest level of weight by early morning, after urinating. Whenever we do experiments, this is when we weigh people, because this is their absolute basal body weight.

Expert consulted
Pamela Peeke, M.D.
Assistant clinical professor of medicine
University of Maryland
Bethesda
Author of Fight Fat after Forty

clogging cholesterol. Instead, plan that 25 percent of your calories come from mono- and polyunsaturated fats, found in fish, olive oil, nuts, and seeds. Studies show that monounsaturated fats, in particular, may reduce your risk of heart disease. So sprinkle nuts and seeds on your salads. Add avocado to your sandwiches. Use olive oil instead of butter for cooking. Keep the portions small; regardless of whether fat is saturated or unsaturated, it still packs 9 calories per gram, compared with carbohydrate and protein's 4.

Eat Early, Eat Often

The best way to lose weight? Eating. It sounds like a Catch-22, but many weight loss experts say that women who want to lose weight first need to learn how to eat. That means breakfast, lunch, and dinner, with a few healthy snacks to keep the edge off.

"Most of us need to replenish our body fuel every 3 to 4 hours," explains Cindy Moore, R.D., director of nutrition therapy at the Cleveland Clinic Foundation and a spokesperson for the American Dietetic Association. "Eating regularly keeps our blood sugar at stable, healthy levels so we stay energized."

It also keeps us motivated to make healthy choices.

"When your blood sugar is low, your willpower is low," Moore says. "That's when you're inclined to eat sweets or foods that are high in fat, like a candy bar, when you're preparing dinner."

"Eating also raises the metabolic rate," adds Cyndi Reeser, R.D., lead nutritionist at the Lipid Research Clinic at George Washington University in Washington, D.C. Just the process of digestion, absorption, and metabolism requires more energy than doing nothing, but when you start dieting, your resting metabolic rate goes down because you're taking in fewer calories. "If you dramatically cut back on calories, your body thinks it's starving," she says, "so it won't burn as many calories while it's resting."

Snacks can help (see The Art of Snacking on page 113 for tips on incorporating healthy snacking into your weight loss plan); so can eating more substantial meals, especially earlier in the day. "Women often eat too lightly during the day and too heavily at night," says Reeser. She suggests reducing calories moderately for best results.

DON'T PUT THIS IN YOUR PANTRY

One bite, and we know we're lost.

As that creamy spoonful of dark chocolate truffle ice cream melts on our tongues, we reach for another. And another. Until the carton is scraped clean, decimating the day's food plans along with our self-esteem. Demoralized, we begin to think that we'll never lose weight.

Nutritionists call ice cream a trigger food for a reason. Depending on our tastes, this frozen treat (as well as its chocolate and cookie cousins) can tempt us to eat far more than we intended, leading to a self-sabotaging cycle of disappointment and overeating. Dietitians refuse to label foods as "good" or "bad," saying that we can eat anything we choose if we eat small quantities. But even they make an exception for trigger foods. When you can't control how much you eat of a particular food, it's the last thing that should be in your pantry.

"If you're a chocoholic and you love pizza, you may not want to include those in your food plan right away, especially not on a day when you're already feeling out of control," says Franca Alphin, R.D., administrative director of the Diet and Fitness Center at Duke University in Durham, North Carolina. "As you learn to manage your eating better, you can slowly add these foods back."

Other common offenders include chips and salty snack foods. But a trigger food can be something as simple as pasta or as comforting as mashed potatoes. Any food you use to make you feel better is a food that you need to watch. "Whatever we have on hand is what we're going to eat, so if we have junk or poor choices, that's what we're going to end up eating," says Mary Martha Smoak, R.D., a registered dietitian at Wake Forest University Baptist Medical Center in Winston-Salem, North Carolina.

To prevent the contents of your pantry from derailing

We need to balance our eating throughout the day, roughly dividing our total calories into fourths: one-fourth each to breakfast, lunch, dinner, and snacks.

your weight loss plans, nutritionists recommend keeping the following items out of our kitchens.

Treats for the kids. "If you have potato chips and cookies in the house for your kids, you're going to eat them, too," warns Laura Molseed, R.D., outpatient nutrition coordinator at the University of Pittsburgh Medical Center. Our sons and daughters don't need the empty calories any more than we do. Consider it a chance to set a healthy example. "Kids do what Mom does," Molseed adds. Do we want them to struggle with their weight, or learn to live healthy lives?

Soft drinks. These sweetened beverages add up to serious calories. Just a 12-ounce can of regular cola contains 152 calories. Drink water instead.

Alcohol. When we drink alcoholic beverages, we don't think of them as caloric, and we forget to factor them into our eating plans. But beer, wine, and liquor contain 7 calories per gram, almost as much as fat. Additionally, when we drink alcoholic beverages, our metabolism responds much as it does when we eat fat. Instead of burning those calories right away, our bodies store them for later use (usually on our thighs and butts). "Women who want to lose weight while continuing to drink alcohol will have a harder time getting the results they want," says Cyndi Reeser, R.D., lead nutritionist at the Lipid Research Clinic at George Washington University in Washington, D.C.

Foods for us, foods for our families. "Don't cook two meals," says Gail Curtis, director of the weight management program at Wake Forest University Baptist Medical Center in Winston-Salem, North Carolina. If your family rebels, she says, pitch it to them this way: "This is something I'm doing for our health. If you don't like what I've prepared, you are free to make something else for yourself."

The changes don't need to come all at once. Think about your own eating habits and daily routine. Perhaps you could nibble on fruit instead of potato chips for your afternoon snack or munch some toast and cheese with your morning cappuccino. Maybe you could bring your lunch a few times a week or eschew the local trattoria in favor of a home-cooked meal Friday nights.

Pick one, says Moore. Stick to it for 2 weeks until it becomes a habit. At the end of the 2 weeks, choose another small change, carefully maintaining your newest healthy eating habit.

Plan Those Meals

By 4:00 P.M. every day, 60 percent of us still have no idea what we're having for dinner. That's a trend we need to change; when we're hungry, tired, and clueless about our next meal, we get into trouble.

But start slowly. Excitedly deciding to make every recipe in your new low-fat cookbook is likely to leave you with a refrigerator full of spoiling food, a pizza delivery boy on your doorstep, and a boatload of frustration. So experts recommend these tips.

Be realistic. When you consider the coming week's menu, ask yourself how often you'll be eating out, when you'll be bringing lunch, and how many nights you'll be able to prepare dinner from scratch, suggests Joan Hammeren, R.D., a registered dietitian at the University of Colorado Health Sciences Center's Weight Choice program in Denver. As you plan your menus, plan your grocery list at the same time.

Keep it simple. Don't stress yourself out by agonizing over every detail of each meal, says Franca Alphin, R.D., administrative director of

TOP TOPS TIP

Make Time for Meals

As a busy mom of two children, Alayne Gunto rarely sat down to eat, especially when she was in the middle of a task. "If I was cleaning house, I never stopped long enough for a meal," says Alayne, 35, who lives in Moundsville, West Virginia. "I'd grab a handful of potato chips and get back to work. I never ate breakfast. By 11:00 A.M., I'd be starving, but I wouldn't eat lunch either. I'd just snatch some crackers or a peanut butter-and-jelly sandwich and keep going."

Her nonstop habits, while keeping her home tidy, had some serious consequences for her figure. When she joined TOPS in 1996, Alayne weighed 235 pounds.

Today, she's 100 pounds slimmer, and a former TOPS "queen" for losing the most weight in her chapter. Her advice on controlling an out-of-control appetite? Eat regular meals and don't leave home without healthy snacks and condiments.

"When I started trying to lose weight, I had to learn to eat three meals a day," Alayne says. Not surprisingly, breakfast was the biggest challenge. Through trial and error, she found that the best time for her morning meal was after her children left for school and her husband went to work. "Now, I sit down at about 9:00 A.M. and eat my breakfast," Alayne says. "Some days, it's oatmeal or raisin bran; other days, I'll have half a bagel or English muffin and some fruit. That's usually enough to tide me over until lunchtime."

Alayne's healthy new habits have carried over to other meals, too. Around 12:30 P.M., she takes time for a light lunch, preparing herself a salad or tuna sandwich. And when she's on the go, this TOPS member travels prepared, carrying pretzels or fruit with her. Should she end up at a restaurant or fast-food joint, she's ready for that, too, with packets of fat-free dressing and fat-free butter spray for seasoning bread, steamed veggies, or popcorn.

the Diet and Fitness Center at Duke University in Durham, North Carolina. Weekly menu planning can be as easy as jotting down a main dish, such as "Monday: chicken" or "Friday: pizza." Fill in the fruits, vegetables, and grains from your well-stocked pantry and freezer.

Go short, go long. None of us has time to hit the supermarket on a daily basis, but we hate monster shopping trips even more. As a compromise, Hammeren suggests making "short shops" once or twice a week to buy just what you need in terms of produce, lean meats, dairy, and lunch items. Save the staples for occasional "big shops."

Stock nonperishables. During those "big shops," buy basics such as canned beans, quick brown rice, pasta, canned green chilies, cous-cous, low-sodium chicken broth, canned tomatoes, and other staples for on-the-fly weeknight dinners, Hammeren recommends. Keep your freezer stocked with frozen vegetables, including chopped onions and peppers and whole grain breads.

Make a list. Is there anything more frustrating than reaching into your cupboard for a quick supper of canned tomatoes and dried pasta only to find that you used the last of them for veggie lasagna the other night? Post a running grocery list on your fridge or inside your organizer. When you're almost out of something, write it down, suggests Hammeren.

Cook in quantities. It's as easy to cook for 12 as it for 6. Just double the recipe. Freeze enough for another meal and use leftovers for lunches.

Back to Basics

So you're planning your menus. What should they consist of?

Real food. Food that still bears some resemblance to its original state. This means fruits and vegetables, whole grains, beans, lean meats, water.

"Anytime you can eat a simple food, like a grilled chicken breast, it'll be lower in calories than fried chicken or chicken with a high-fat sauce," says Mary Martha Smoak, R.D., a registered dietitian at Wake Forest University Baptist Medical Center in Winston-Salem, North Carolina. Unprocessed foods also have more naturally occurring nutrients, including various vitamins, minerals, and fiber and less added sodium, sugar, and fat.

Here's how to reorient your meals toward natural choices.

Drink water. Cold and calorie-free, water is your best friend in your lifestyle change. Choose it over soda, sweetened fruit drinks, and sweetened tea as often as you can, and you could lose up to 1 pound a week, says Dr. Chauncey.

It's not that you'll eat less, for contrary to a common weight loss myth, water doesn't fill you up. But you won't be adding extra calories from a nonfilling liquid either, says Smoak. Some women discover through food diaries that they drank as many as 1,000 calories a day without feeling full from the liquid.

You'll also stay well-hydrated. "Women often drink too little water," Reeser says. "They forget the role that fluid balance plays in weight reduction and general health."

To liven up your eight daily glasses, have it over ice with a twist of lemon or lime. Can't stand the chemical taste of tap water? Use filtered pitchers or splurge for bottled. Choose calorie-free carbonated waters for a fizzy treat, drink unsweetened herbal teas hot or cold, and dilute your favorite juice with water for a low-calorie thirst quencher.

Look for whole grains. By eating whole grain breads, cereals, and pastas, you'll boost your fiber intake, filling your stomach while you trim calories. But remember, just because a bread isn't white doesn't mean it has a lot of fiber in it. Brown bread, for example, may get its coloring from caramel coloring. Read food labels carefully. You want "whole grains" listed as one of the top ingredients, says Dr. O'Shaughnessy.

Other good sources include barley, whole wheat couscous, and brown and wild rice, says Moore. For noodle lovers, many supermarkets now carry whole wheat pasta. If your family is new to whole grain pasta, start slowly. Mix one part whole grain noodles to two parts regular, upping the whole grain proportions as you become adjusted to the taste and higher fiber content.

Learn to love beans. High in protein, dried beans and other legumes should be a staple in your diet. They're a meat substitute for vegetarians as well as a healthy complement to beef, chicken, and fish.

Filled with fiber, beans and lentils break down slowly in your body, keeping your stomach full longer and your blood sugar levels stable, says Laura Molseed, R.D., outpatient nutrition coordinator at the University of Pittsburgh Medical Center. This sends a one-two knockout punch to temptation when the office pastry cart appears or you pass a vending machine.

Forget the soak-overnight-and-cook-for-3-hours beans. Today's canned beans (rinse them to eliminate most of the sodium) go nicely in

WOMAN TO WOMAN

She Learned That Fat-Free Foods Weren't the Answer

Every January, Susan Cursi of Fresno, California, had the same New Year's resolution: Lose weight. Yet she gained and gained, adding about 10 pounds annually to her 5-foot-5-inch frame until she hit 190 pounds in 1993 and decided that she'd had enough. She began eating fat-free foods, but found them full of empty calories and empty promises. Seven years later, Susan, now 51, weighs 130 pounds and serves as a national spokeswoman for TOPS. Here is her story.

When I started trying to lose weight, I began eating more fat-free products. I bought fat-free mayonnaise, fat-free sour cream, fat-free cheeses. But it wasn't satisfying. With some fat-free products, the carton probably tastes better than the food. Try to make a pizza with fat-free cheese—let me tell you, it doesn't work.

I found that I started losing the most weight when I just started eating sensibly. I chose foods that I liked, but I ate smaller quantities. I watched my portion size and ate only until I was satisfied, not stuffed. I learned how to incorporate fat back into my food plan so that I could continue losing weight while feeling satisfied with what I was eating.

Today, I use the reduced-fat versions of products, such as light sour cream or ice cream. You don't get as many fat grams, and it still tastes good. When I want a cookie, I go to a great bakery and buy just one. If you buy a package of fat-free cookies, you'll end up eating several—if not the entire box. If I'm going to spend my calories on a cookie, I want it to be the best.

But she cautions women with diabetes to check with their doctors before eating large portions of certain fruits.

If getting the recommended five-a-day sounds about as likely as your teenager awakening before noon on a Saturday, have faith (and follow these simple tips).

- Remember the saying, "out of sight, out of mind"? That goes double for fruit. If you're lucky enough to be in the market for a new refrigerator, look for one with clear shelves and drawers so that you can see what's hiding behind the milk. Otherwise, post a list of just-purchased fruit on the refrigerator door or keep your fruit in a pretty bowl or basket on the counter. Apply the same principle at work. If you bring grapes for a snack, don't leave them to bruise in your briefcase or turn into gray glop in the refrigerator. Put them on your desk for mindful munching.
- For the best taste and prices on fresh produce, learn what the best seasons are for fruit. Somehow a cantaloupe in January just isn't going to have that sweet-as-sugar taste as one eaten in July. You'll also save if you purchase just what you know you'll eat. Live alone? You don't need an entire box of clementines; just a few naval oranges will do nicely. Finally, don't forget about canned and frozen fruits. Look for fruits canned in light syrup or their own juices; they're lower in calories.

salads, spaghetti sauces, and casseroles. Lentils are another option; they cook faster.

Finagle more fruits. Low in calories and high in nutrients, fruit qualifies as a dietary mainstay of many university weight management programs. Dr. Chauncey tells her female patients to eat as much fruit as they want. It's healthy and it keeps the hunger pangs at bay.

Venerate veggies. Whether you like them steamed or stir-fried, roasted or raw, vegetables should be the mainstay on your plate. From the calcium in broccoli to the lycopene in tomatoes, veggies contain vitamins, minerals, and phytonutrients essential to our health, no matter what we weigh.

Like fruit, vegetables satisfy with minimal calories, providing about 3 grams of fiber per serving, cooked or raw. To get more into your diet, stir chopped veggies into spaghetti sauce. Add sprouts or lettuce and tomato to sandwiches. Eat yams for snacks, cutting an x in the top and microwaving on high for 10 to 12 minutes, or until tender. Look for packages of baby carrots, prewashed mixed greens, and ready-to-go salads.

"Buying already prepared vegetables may seem expensive, but if you eat them, they're worth it," says Suzanne W. Dixon, R.D., a research epidemiologist and registered dietitian at the Henry Ford Health System in Detroit.

Got milk? "Women do not drink enough milk," says Dr. O'Shaughnessy, who treats women for osteoporosis. "They're worried about the extra calories, and it's not as convenient as a diet soda from the office vending machine."

Instead, milk may be a weight loss catalyst.

When researchers followed women for 2 years, they discovered that those who ate less than 1,900 calories and consumed at least 1,000 milligrams of calcium daily—primarily from fat-free milk, yogurt, and regular cheese—lost 6 pounds of body fat. Women who took in fewer than 500 milligrams of calcium gained 2 to 3 pounds of body fat.

WOMEN ASK WHY

What's calorie density, and why should I care?

Very simply, calorie density is the amount of calories in a food, expressed per gram of weight. Generally, the more fat a food contains, the more calorie-dense it is.

Oil, for example, is all fat, so it tops the calorie density list. But a whole cup of raw spinach, with virtually no fat, has the lowest calorie density. So if you want the most volume of food that will still let you lose weight, look for things that give you the largest portions with the fewest calories.

Expert consulted
Roxanne E. Moore, R.D.
Nutrition education coordinator
Towson University
Baltimore

To get your daily calcium, try 1 cup of low-fat cottage cheese (400 milligrams), 8 ounces of fat-free milk (300 milligrams), a cup of low-fat yogurt (350 milligrams) and ½ cup fat-free frozen yogurt (50 milligrams).

Break the Fast

Women, notorious breakfast skippers in the best of nutritional times, are even worse when trying to lose weight, says Molseed. In a misguided attempt to cut calories, we skip the first meal of the day with disastrous consequences for our diets.

"It only ends up making you hungrier later," Molseed says. In contrast, when you start your day with a small meal, you may be less likely to overeat at later meals because you won't feel so ravenous, says Hammeren.

For a morning meal that keeps you going until lunch, combine carbohydrates, like oatmeal or high-fiber, ready-to-eat cereal or whole wheat breads, with lean protein, like low-fat milk, yogurt, or scrambled eggs made with egg substitute, suggests Hammeren.

Breakfast is also the perfect meal to begin sneaking in servings of fruit, says Alphin. Sprinkle fresh or frozen blueberries over cereal, stir raisins into oatmeal, or mix thawed frozen strawberries into yogurt.

If you can't remember the last time your day started with more than a low-fat latte-to-go, give these tips a try.

Say hello to cereal. With fat-free milk, it's low-fat and low-fuss. Check the nutrition information before you buy; you want a cereal with no more than 14 grams of sugar per serving and at least 7 grams of fiber. "If you eat something very sweet at breakfast, you'll set yourself up for more sweets later when your blood sugar crashes," Alphin says. If you can't live without Cap'n Crunch, mix it with a high-fiber variety like Post Raisin Bran or Kellogg's All-Bran.

Think liquid. No time to sit and eat? Take it with you. Blend 1 cup fat-free milk with half a frozen banana, 1 teaspoon sugar, 1 cup frozen strawberries, and enough soy powder to equal 7 grams of protein for a sweet, creamy smoothie.

Get toasted. The protein-carb combo of peanut butter or low-fat cream cheese on a slice of whole wheat toast, an English muffin, or half a bagel will start your day off right.

Go portable. Stock your fridge with hard-boiled eggs, cartons of yogurt, and sliced cheese that you can slap on some bread and take with you for breakfast on the run. If you have an extra few minutes, stir 1/4 cup of Grape-Nuts cereal into yogurt for extra crunch and fiber.

Remember old favorites. On a chilly morning, oatmeal makes a comforting, high-fiber breakfast. Combine 1/2 cup of oats with 1 cup fat-free milk, one apple (chopped and unpeeled), 2 tablespoons wheat germ, and 2 teaspoons brown sugar and cook according to package directions.

Beat the clock. If the smell of scrambled eggs in the morning makes you burrow under the bedcovers, skip breakfast in favor of brunch. Before the clock strikes noon, eat a piece of fruit, a slice of toast, a stick of string cheese, or low-fat yogurt, says Hammeren.

Eat lightly at night. Just not hungry in the mornings? Eat less in the evenings. "It's best to curb food intake at night, when metabolism slows," Reeser says. "Do whatever it takes to keep your hands busy. Make crafts. Write. If you have to go to bed to avoid eating, go to bed. You'll be hungrier in the mornings." Then you can eat that oh-so-good-for-you breakfast.

Go for Low Energy Density

For Barbara Rolls, Ph.D., co-author of *Volumetrics: Feel Full on Fewer Calories*, the key to losing weight isn't just calories or fat grams but also "energy density." Basically, energy density is affected by how much water a food contains. The higher the water content, the lower the energy density. The lower the energy density, the fuller you'll feel on fewer calories.

Also, the more fat in a food, the higher its energy density because fat packs a lot of calories into a small amount of food, says Dr. Rolls, who is also the Guthrie Chair of Nutrition at Pennsylvania State University in University Park.

Dry and high in fat, potato chips qualify as high-energy density food, while broth-based vegetable soup is low, helped by the high water content of the broth and vegetables.

Even if we've never heard of the concept, energy density influences how much we eat. "Day after day, people tend to eat a constant weight or volume of food because they've learned how much usually satisfies them," Dr. Rolls says. For instance, you're going to eat three slices of pizza, whether it has sausage or vegetables on it. But if you ordered the one with vegetables, you'd be just as full on far fewer calories. So, she says, since you're going to be eating the same amount, make sure that what you're eating is low energy density so that it will also be low in calories.

Energy density can also trip us up when we're trying to lose weight. "When women diet, they start eating tiny portions," Dr. Rolls says. "They haven't learned that it's important to fill their plates for visual and physical reasons." Those tiny portions will just leave us aching for more food. When you choose foods low in energy density, however, such as strawberries or spinach, you can eat enough to fill you up yet not worry about high calories, she says.

Here's how you can lower the energy density of your meals.

Add extra vegetables to entrées. Instead of a cup of pasta with a ½ cup of Alfredo sauce, toss a cup of cooked pasta with tomatoes, summer squash, mushrooms, broccoli, olive oil, Parmesan cheese, and herbs. For the same calories, you'll be able to eat 3½ cups of pasta primavera versus 1½ cups of the Alfredo. Also try adding grapes and apples to chicken salad or pile veggies on pizza.

Slurp soup. With their high water content, broth-based soups are the queen of low energy density foods. When Dr. Rolls served women soup for lunch, they ate fewer calories at lunch and didn't make up for them at dinner, compared with those who dined on an equally caloric

CALORIE DENSITIES: A BAKER'S DOZEN

Here are 13 common food items and quantities, their calories, and their calories per gram.

Food	Calories per Serving	Calories per Gram
Oil (1 Tbsp)	120	8.8
Cheese nachos (7 oz)	615	3.1
Glazed doughnut (2 oz)	240	4.3
French fries (large; 6 oz)	578	3.4
Tuna salad sandwich (11 oz)	718	2.3
Grilled chicken (6 oz)	270	1.5
Broiled flounder (6 oz)	200	1.2
Baked potato with skin	220	1.1
Low-fat fruit yogurt (8 oz)	243	1.0
One apple (medium)	81	0.6
One raw carrot (large)	30	0.4
Cooked broccoli (½ cup)	22	0.3
Raw spinach (1 cup)	6	0.2

casserole accompanied by a glass of water. Take advantage of these effects when you're eating out by ordering broth-based (not cream-based) soup as an appetizer.

Start with salad. An appetizer salad of leafy greens will take the edge off your appetite before your higher-calorie entrée arrives. To keep the meal's energy density down, use less regular dressing, or use fat-free dressing instead.

Choose fresh fruits over dried. If you have trouble eating fresh produce before it spoils, dried fruits are the perfect answer. But their high energy density means that a little box of raisins goes a long way calorie-wise. When you're starving at 3:00 P.M., 2 cups of grapes are more filling than ¼ cup of raisins, with the same number of calories.

Calories Do Count

You've trimmed the fat in your breakfasts, lunches, and dinners. You're eating foods that have low energy density. You're snacking on fruits and veggies. But the pounds still aren't melting away. Perhaps it's time to look at your overall calories.

"With many women who are struggling to lose weight, it's not so much the makeup of their meals but how much they're eating," says Hammeren.

Trim 200 to 500 calories each day—about the equivalent of a couple of sodas and a piece of cheesecake. Just be sure that your overall calorie count doesn't drop below 1,200, or you'll miss out on vital nutrients, says Curtis.

Add enough exercise to burn another 250 calories daily—about 45 minutes of brisk walking (see The Way You Do the Things You Do on page 91 and We Can Work It Out on page 100 for suggestions)—and you'll lose roughly 1 to 2 pounds a week. It sounds like slow going, but it works.

"We understand you want to lose the weight yesterday," says Curtis. "But you have to remember that you didn't gain it yesterday."

To cut calories, you don't need to eliminate foods; just control portion sizes.

But what is a portion, anyway? "Some people seem to think that a portion is whatever they eat or whatever they're served," Smoak says. The answer is far more precise. For instance, 1 cup of leafy raw vegetables (such as spinach or romaine lettuce), ½ cup of cooked or raw veggies (such as carrots or cooked spinach), and ½ cup of cooked legumes all qualify as a portion of vegetables.

A serving of fruit? That would be ¾ cup of juice—not the tumblerful of orange drink that we down each morning. The same goes for bagels. Halve that chunk of boiled bread, and you have a serving, according to the USDA.

But even dietitians admit that measuring food gets tedious fast. So they recommend trying these shortcuts.

Test yourself. Get out your favorite cereal bowl, coffee cup, and juice glass. Fill them with the quantity of food and drinks that you normally have. Then pour their contents into measuring cups. How does your morning bowl of cereal compare with the recommended serving size on the packages? How many servings are you actually eating? If you discover that you're drinking 1½ cups of apple juice every morning, trade half those liquid calories for an apple. You'll get more stomach-filling fiber, and your blood sugar levels will stay more stable than if you just drank the juice alone.

Watch proportions. For a well-balanced meal that supports your weight loss, divide your dinner plate into quarters. Allocate one-quarter for lean protein, one-half for vegetables or fruits, and one-quarter for grains. "Women overcarb it," says Pamela Peeke, M.D., assistant clinical professor of medicine at the University of Maryland in Bethesda and author of *Fight Fat after Forty*. "Men overprotein it. They eat a hunk of steak. We eat a hunk of bagel." As we age, our metabolism slows down, and we no longer need all the energy contained in starchy foods such as pasta, rice, potatoes, and breads, Dr. Peeke says. Treat carbohydrates like a treat, especially at dinnertime, basing your meals on veggies and fruit instead.

Use smaller dishes. Your petite plates and bowls will look satisfying and full even with smaller portions.

Check your temptations. We can never eat too many fruits and vegetables, but it's easy to overdo other luscious foods. If you suspect that you're overeating certain foods, grab your measuring cup and find out. You don't have to give up the blueberry muffin from the neighborhood bakery, but you should know how many servings it constitutes and how many calories and fat grams it contributes to your day. Then you can occasionally work it into your food plan.

Don't eat out of containers. "I find it very hard to monitor how many chips I've eaten when I'm just dipping my hand into the bag," Reeser admits. So pour out a portion, reseal the package, and put it away.

Indulge Yourself

Chocolate chip cookie dough. Sour cream and onion potato chips. Mashed potatoes with real butter. Whether our tastes tend toward sweet, sour, or salty, we all have culinary indulgences that we refuse to live without, no matter how many pounds we want to lose.

And we don't have to. "If you really want a Snickers bar every day, then plan it in," Alphin says.

There will be trade-offs, however. You may not be able to eat both the Snickers bar and the potato chips every day, or an entire pint of ice cream at one sitting. But you don't need to deny yourself foods that you genuinely relish in the name of weight loss. Such a rigid approach to eating makes you feel deprived and rebellious. So if you're eating nothing but spinach salad for a week straight, sooner or later, you're going to have a Fritos binge, blindly munching chip after chip until nothing is left but the salt that you're licking off your fingers.

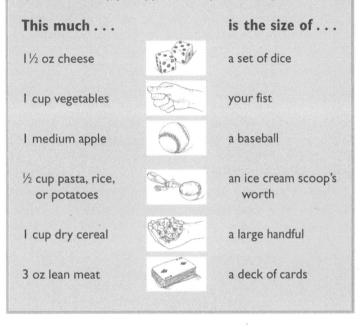

WHAT'S A PORTION?

Not knowing at a glance what constitutes ounces or cups can make portion control a guessing game. The next time you're without your measuring cups, think of the items in this chart to help you approximate your serving sizes.

This much . . .		is the size of . . .
1½ oz cheese		a set of dice
1 cup vegetables		your fist
1 medium apple		a baseball
½ cup pasta, rice, or potatoes		an ice cream scoop's worth
1 cup dry cereal		a large handful
3 oz lean meat		a deck of cards

Instead, incorporate small, edible pleasures into each day. "Food should be pleasurable," says Judith S. Stern, R.D., Sc.D., professor of nutrition and internal medicine at the University of California, Davis. "We all want to eat and enjoy it, but no one wants their lives to be ruled by it."

So try this.

Indulge only in what you love. When Alphin recommends changes to her women patients' eating habits, she often hears, "I never really liked that anyhow." If a sliver of cheesecake is what makes your heart beat faster, don't waste those calories on kettle-cooked potato chips.

Time your treats. Give in to your sweet cravings when you're least likely to overeat, Dr. Stern advises. If a week without ice cream is like

Christmas without Santa, order it in small amounts for dessert when you're dining at a restaurant. That way, you won't be standing in front of your refrigerator scooping it out of the carton.

Buy small quantities. When we purchase jumbo packages, we end up eating jumbo-size portions. Researchers at the University of Illinois at Urbana–Champaign found that people ate between 7 to 43 percent more food when serving themselves from larger containers. That's not a problem if you're buying a bushel of apples, but it will be if your grocery cart is stuffed with family-size bags of cheese doodles. Purchase single-serving packages of sweet or salty treats. If it's ice cream you love, buy pints or ice-cream bars rather than half-gallons.

Make it a ritual. Create a ceremony to revel in your favorite food pleasures. Serve ice cream in ramekins with delicate spoons after dinner. Use your best china for French fries. You'll eat more slowly and enjoy every bite.

Consider substitutes. Save fat and calories by looking for lighter versions of food luxuries. Choose baked tortilla chips instead of fried, sorbet over full-fat ice cream, diet soda instead of regular. Just don't devour the entire package, thinking that "fat-free" means "calorie-free." Many fat-free items are just as high in sugar and calories as their regular counterparts.

Go for the real thing. Substitutes don't always satisfy. If you hate the taste of low-fat cheese, for example, buy the real stuff and eat it in small, flavorful quantities that give you as much taste per calorie as possible. When you control your portion size, no food is forbidden indefinitely, says Hammeren.

The Way You Do the Things You Do: How Activity Burns Fat

Why spend hundreds of dollars on expensive exercise equipment when you can get the same calorie burn with a broom, a dustpan, and a warren of dust bunnies?

That's right. Housework burns fat. Until recently, it seemed that the only way to solve the *burn more calories* part of the weight loss equation was to sweat it out at the gym for an hour or so several times a week. Not so. Research shows that moderate activity can burn fat just as efficiently as a structured exercise program.

So what exactly qualifies as moderate-intensity activity?

On the effort scale, moderate would rate the equivalent of a brisk walk. That's about as fast as you might walk if you were late for an appointment or trying to catch a bus, says Bess H. Marcus, Ph.D., associate professor of psychiatry and human behavior at the Brown University Center for Behavioral and Preventive Medicine in Providence, Rhode Island. It's not a stroll through the mall.

One study, called Project Active, conducted at the Cooper Institute for Aerobics Research in Dallas, compared two ways of getting 235 sedentary men and women moving. Half the participants were instructed to work out in a gym for 30 minutes at least three times a week. The other half met one night a week in small groups to discuss ways to integrate physical activity into their lives.

Instead of going to the gym, the lifestyle group found ways to use the stairs more often, walk farther to restrooms, and generally make life a little more labor-intensive. "People got real creative about how to work more activity into their lives. Physical activity was suddenly on their radar screen," says Dr. Marcus, who was one of the co-authors of the study.

After just 6 months, both groups had comparable increases in physical activity, using up about 150 extra calories a day. That's the equivalent of about 30 minutes of moderate-intensity activity—all you need to start burning fat.

Every Step Counts

Instead of thinking of exercise as pain and sweat, think of it as your body in motion—any kind of motion. Or to put it another way: The

BURNIN' CALORIES

If you are a 150-pound woman, how long does it take to burn 150 more calories a day? That depends on what you do. (If you weigh more, it may take less intensity to burn the same amount of calories.)

Ironing	59 minutes
Cooking	48 minutes
Washing and waxing a car	45 to 60 minutes
Playing volleyball	45 minutes
Strolling through the mall	44 minutes
Grocery shopping	36 minutes
Doing yoga	36 minutes
Vacuuming	34 minutes
Playing horseshoes	33 minutes
Gardening	30 to 45 minutes
Bicycling leisurely	5 miles in 30 minutes
Brisk walking	30 minutes
Dancing fast	30 minutes
Pushing a stroller	30 minutes
Raking leaves	30 minutes
Mowing the lawn with a power push mower	29 minutes
Inline skating leisurely	26 minutes
Stacking firewood	25 minutes
Bowling	23 minutes
Housecleaning	21 minutes
Scrubbing floors	20 minutes
Swimming	19 minutes
Climbing stairs	15 minutes
Shoveling snow	15 minutes

and too little moving. Blame our harried schedules or the conveniences of modern technology. With the click of a switch, we can open a garage door, change the channel on the TV, or go shopping all over the globe. All in all, fewer than one in four of us gets the 30 minutes of daily activity recommended by health experts. That's a lot of unspent calories.

"Basically, at the turn of the 20th century, something like 85 percent of our workforce worked in agricultural-related jobs," says Barbara Moore, Ph.D., president of Shape Up America!, in Washington, D.C. "They were very physically demanding. In today's information-based society, so much of the work we do requires sitting and only sitting."

According to a study from the United Kingdom, people there burn about 800 calories less per day than they did in 1970, mostly because of automation and labor-saving devices. It's the same story on this side of the Atlantic.

"Physical activity has been pushed out of our lives," says Miriam Nelson, Ph.D., associate chief of the Human Physiology Laboratory at the Jean Mayer USDA Human Nutrition Research Center on Aging at Tufts University in Boston and author of *Strong Women Stay Slim.* "This means we have to choose ways to work activity back into our lives. We have to consciously get up more, walk more, take the stairs more. Whenever possible, we need to seek out activity."

more you move your arms and legs, the more calories you burn. The more you sit or lie still, the fewer calories you burn.

The problem is, we're doing too much sitting

Most moderate-intensity activities—walking briskly, raking leaves, mowing the lawn with a push mower, or vacuuming—will burn 150 calories in about 30 minutes. So instead of just counting calories, also add up your minutes of activity each day. To lose weight and keep it off, you actually need about 60 minutes of activity a day, according to the latest research.

It doesn't make any difference if you do it all at once or break it up into smaller chunks of time. "Everything counts," says Dr. Moore.

Step up the intensity. Michelle Edwards, a health educator and certified personal trainer at the Cooper Institute, advises her clients to start by simply increasing the intensity of any physical activity that they're already doing. That can mean taking the stairs a little faster, choosing parking spots at the far end of the lot, or making wider arm circles when wiping off the kitchen counter. The idea is to put a little more effort into every activity in order to burn more calories.

Keep a diary. For the next few days, clock yourself every time you walk, clean, garden, climb a flight of stairs, or perform any other activity that involves moving the muscles in your arms and legs. At the end of the day, add up your active time. It helps create a vivid picture of how the minutes add up, explains Edwards. Once you do this, you'll probably find yourself thinking of all kinds of ways to add a few more minutes here and there throughout the day.

One of the keys to becoming more active is learning to identify opportunities in your day and taking advantage of them. "Five minutes

---

Does Thriller TV Burn More Calories?

Park yourself in front of the television for some well-deserved down time, and you'll burn a measly 27 calories per sit-com. But what about those times when you're riveted to a heart-racing, teeth-clenching Stephen King thriller? Do you burn more calories?

Researchers in England at the University of Newcastle on Tyne decided to find out. They had a dozen people fast overnight and then watch various movies such as *Alien* and *Death on the Nile*. They tested how many calories they burned by measuring heart rate, respiration, and body temperature.

It turns out that no matter how exciting the programming is, as long as you're sitting, you won't burn any extra calories. Even so, watching TV doesn't have to be a totally listless experience, says Michelle Edwards, a health educator and certified personal trainer at the Cooper Institute for Aerobics Research in Dallas.

Instead of staying put during commercials, stand up and walk in place, do jumping jacks, skip rope, or just dance, says Edwards. The average adult watches about 22 hours of TV a week. Considering that the average hour-long prime-time drama has about 20 minutes of commercials, that adds up to a whopping 440 minutes of potential activity a week. Now who says they don't have time to exercise?

---

here; ten minutes there. It all adds up," says Edwards.

It also helps to record how much time you spend sitting each day, and to do the reverse. Figure out ways to gradually replace the sitting with activity.

Get a pedometer. If you want to get a clearer picture of the amount of physical activity you are doing in a day, record how many steps you take on an average day and then find ways to add more. Studies show that people who are active for 30 minutes each day accumulate about

10,000 steps, while the average person who works in an office typically takes about 2,000 to 4,000 steps a day. "A pedometer can be a very motivational tool, a way to self-monitor," says Edwards. "And we know from experience that people who self-monitor are more likely to reach their activity goals than people who do not."

Be prepared. Keep walking shoes in your car or desk so that you can walk whenever you have a few minutes.

Schedule it. We tend to keep our appointments, so make an appointment to exercise. You can start by scheduling exercise in the morning instead of later in the day, suggests Denise Bruner, M.D., president of the American Society of Bariatric Physicians (a group of doctors who specialize in weight loss treatments) and a physician practicing in Arlington, Virginia. "Women seem to be more successful in general if they put activity on the front end of the day versus the end of the day, when either work-related issues or home issues can end up taking precedence over exercise time," she says.

Working Activity In at Work

Besides sleeping, many of us spend the biggest chunk of our time at work. If you can work in three 10-minute walks over the course of your day, you'll burn an extra 150 calories. In a year, that adds up to more than 10 pounds of fat-burning calories. Here's how you can work in a workout.

REAL-LIFE SCENARIO

She Eats Healthy Foods and Exercises, but Still Can't Lose Weight

Madeline, 40, has a great job as a system analyst for a large investment corporation, but as well as her career has been going, she's getting concerned over another aspect of her life: her weight. Over the past 5 years, her weight has crept from about 135 to almost 150 pounds, and nothing she does seems to take off those 15 pounds. Although she often skips lunch, she tries to eat regular meals, and she's careful to eat only low-fat, low-sugar products. Since she spends nearly 9 hours a day sitting at a computer, she also makes sure she keeps lots of water and healthy snacks on hand at work so that she won't binge from hunger when she gets home at night. She also goes to the gym 3 days a week, where she spends 20 minutes on the treadmill. Why can't she lose weight?

Madeline is like most women who experience stubborn weight gain in their thirties. She's not burning enough calories from daily, consistent physical activity. Nine hours behind a desk working on the computer burns up a paltry 50 calories an hour. In order to lose weight, she's going to have to make a conscious effort to increase her daily energy expenditure by at least 250 calories and decrease the number of calories she eats by 250 calories per day.

While Madeline's 60 minutes on the treadmill each week is a good start, it's not enough to have an impact on her weight. On those days when she heads to the gym, she should aim for 30 to 45 minutes of aerobic exercise.

She's also going to need to come up with some time in the regular course of her day when she can become more ac-

Park on the outskirts. As in most cities, parking is scarce in Boston. Dr. Nelson ends up parking about eight blocks from her office each day. But instead of taking the university-provided shuttle, she walks the rest of the way. "I get an eight-minute walk every morning and afternoon. Then I add in a little bit here and there, tive, whether it's her lunch hour, before work, or after work. That might mean making a commitment to taking the stairs instead of the elevator at work. Or, if she uses public transportation, she could get off a few stops early and walk a longer distance.

Finally, Madeline could also begin to strength-train two or three times a week. That would be really helpful in revving up her metabolism.

The flip side of the weight loss equation is how much she's eating. She won't lose weight unless her calorie intake is consistently less than her calorie expenditure.

Madeline seems to be taking a sensible approach to eating, but she's probably still consuming too many calories. Her goal should be to shave about 250 calories a day from her diet, but I wouldn't recommend that she do it by skipping meals. That can slow the body's metabolism and thwart weight loss efforts. She should check the calorie content of the low-fat foods she's been eating to make sure they are also low-calorie. Many women consume these products freely and wonder why they don't lose weight. A better approach is to eat a healthy variety of fruits, vegetables, whole grains and low-fat protein that will provide the nutrients she needs to feel energetic and alert throughout the day.

Expert consulted
Miriam Nelson, Ph.D.
Associate Chief of the Human Physiology
Laboratory
Jean Mayer USDA Human Nutrition Research
Center on Aging at Tufts University
Boston
Author of Strong Women Stay Slim

Take advantage of the speakerphone. Walk around or do stretches while you're on the phone, says Dr. Moore. Standing burns about 30 percent more calories than sitting.

Seek out the stairs instead of the elevator. "Buildings are designed so that the elevator is prominent and the stairs are not," says Dr. Moore. Stairways are tucked away in the far corners of the building and may not seem accessible. Seek them out. "Every opportunity should be seized to take a few steps." If you work in a high-rise, get off the elevator a few floors early and take the stairs the rest of the way. Add more floors as you build stamina.

Schedule a mobile meeting. Instead of sitting in a conference room and meeting over a cup of coffee, schedule a walking meeting.

Take the long way around. Whenever you're walking somewhere, take the long route, whether you're headed to the mail room or the conference room, says Dr. Nelson. Remember, every extra minute of walking burns about 5 calories.

Use the restroom on another floor. Or, if you work in a one-story building, use the restroom farthest away from your desk.

Set an activity timer. Program your computer or watch to remind you to take a brief walk, says Dr. Marcus. Some of the people in the Project Active study set their watches to go off each hour to remind them to take a 5-minute walk. At the end of the workday, they had accumulated 30 to 40 minutes of activity.

Order out. Build activity into your lunch hour. Instead of using the entire hour or half-

and before you know it, I've burned a fair number of calories," she says.

Change your bus stop. If you ride public transportation, you probably already do a fair amount of walking. If you want to add a few more steps to your day, Dr. Moore recommends getting off your mode of transit a few stops early.

WHAT'S A FIDGET?

We all know one—a shapely sylph type who can eat whatever she wants and not gain an ounce, while for the rest of us, just looking at a slice of chocolate cake will attach it firmly to our hips. At long last, researchers at the Mayo Clinic in Rochester, Minnesota, have uncovered a clue to unravel this mystery.

It turns out that some people burn up excess calories from overeating through everyday activities such as changing posture, tapping their feet, moving around—in other words, fidgeting. Researchers call this ability to burn calories NEAT (non-exercise activity thermogenesis).

For 2 months, Mayo Clinic researchers fed 16 normal-weight people an extra 1,000 calories a day—the caloric equivalent of two Big Macs per day. Then they tracked whether the calories were burned or stored as fat or lean tissue.

The amount of weight that the participants gained varied from 2 to 16 pounds. The reason for the difference: The number of calories they burned through NEAT. While some people burned fewer than 100 calories a day, others burned nearly 700 calories.

The message from this study is an optimistic one: Every calorie that you burn by moving around counts. And although NEAT is probably something you do unconsciously, researchers speculate that you may be able to train yourself to increase NEAT by using behavioral cues, such as putting music on while you're doing dishes and moving to the beat.

Activate Your Everyday Life

Our harried home lives often feel anything but inactive. We're constantly on the go from the moment our feet hit the floor in the morning until the last chore is done at night. Who has time to squeeze one more thing onto their to-do list? The good news is that you don't have to do more; you just need to do it differently. You can find hidden opportunities for exercise simply by changing your approach to everyday chores and errands.

Don't let things pile up when you pick up. Eliminate using the bottom stairs as a holding area for stuff that needs to go on another floor, says Dr. Moore. Walk up and down the stairs every time you come across something that needs to be put away.

Walk and talk. Don't settle into your favorite chair for a good, long tête à tête when your best friend calls. Take advantage of the mobility you get using the cordless phone. Walk around, put away odds and ends, or go up and down the stairs while you talk.

Be an active captive. From women in the Project Active study, researchers heard a lot about having to take their kids places. "Think if there is some way for *you* to get more activity while you're a captive at your child's activities," says Dr. Marcus. Walk around the soccer field while watching the game. Take a walk around the block during the half-hour piano lesson.

Get lean while you clean. We're spending about 18 hours a week doing housework—half

hour to eat, save at least 10 minutes for a brisk walk. Or, you could try ordering your lunch from a restaurant that's six blocks away instead of one that's right around the corner, and then walk to get it, says Dr. Nelson.

Never take the escalator down. No, you don't burn as many calories walking down the steps as you do going up, but it's still an opportunity to move those muscles, says Dr. Moore. To boost your burn, swing your arms as you're walking down the stairs or downhill.

the time that our mothers spent. "I always recommend that people do housework to boost their activity level," says Dr. Moore. We're not suggesting you step back into the days of domestic drudgery, but when you do clean, use large, exaggerated movements, and you'll burn more calories.

Do your own yard work. No more hiring a neighborhood kid to rake leaves or cut grass. Do an hour of yard work a week, and you'll burn about 300 extra calories. But don't use a power mower. "If you do, you won't burn 300 calories of your fat. You'll burn gasoline instead," says Dr. Moore.

Tote more groceries. It seems much more efficient to try and lug every single bag of groceries into the house in one trip. But you can burn more calories if you make multiple trips and bring the bags in one at a time, says Dr. Moore.

Go back to basics. Find places in your day where you can do a task in a more manual way, says Dr. Nelson. Get out the hose and wash your car yourself instead of taking it to the car wash. Lose your remote control and get up off the couch to switch channels. Walk to the store for a gallon of milk.

GUILT-FREE PLEASURE
Sauna Baths

Anyone who has experienced the pure relief of stepping into an air-conditioned room on a blistering summer day may puzzle over the allure of a sauna bath.

Strange as it may sound to our modern-day American sensibilities, people have sought out the health benefits of a good sweat for thousands of years. Throughout history, doctors have extolled the medicinal value of the sweat bath in its many forms—the Finnish sauna, Russian banai, Islamic hammam, and the Native American sweat lodge.

The basic sauna as we know it today—a log- or wood-paneled room with a rock-filled heater—was developed by Scandinavians more than 1,000 years ago. The first sauna in North America was built before the American Revolution in 1638 by Finnish immigrants who settled near the Delaware River.

In our high-tech, climate-controlled world, this ancient technique of alternating hot air and cold water to cleanse the body can be a perfect way to relax, relieve tension and anxiety, improve circulation, and burn some calories.

When you take a sauna (pronounced "sow-na," not saw-na), the heat hastens circulation, brings bloodflow to the skin, and stimulates sweating.

While you're sitting back taking in the heat, the increased circulation and sweat response burn extra calories. During a half-hour sauna, you can expect to lose roughly 1 to 2 pounds of fluid. Each pound of sweat loss represents 263 calories of dissipated heat.

If you are pregnant or have diabetes, multiple sclerosis or high or low blood pressure, seek the advice of your physician before using a sauna.

PART THREE

The
Minor Keys
of Success

We Can Work It Out: Exercise as an Option

Now hold on a minute! Just because you can get a great calorie burn from all your daily activities doesn't mean that exercise isn't a good idea.

If you put aside some time to do a regular workout, you'll torch even more calories, and your energy and fitness levels should increase, says Lois Sheldahl, Ph.D., associate professor of medicine at the Medical College of Wisconsin and director of the cardiopulmonary rehabilitation center at the Veterans Administration Medical Center in Milwaukee. "Fitting exercise into a busy schedule can make such a big difference in the number of calories you burn each day. You'll be able to lose weight faster or just find it easier to maintain your figure," she says.

And remember, exercise offers benefits that go far beyond weight loss—including increased energy, protection against heart disease and diabetes, and a reduced risk of osteoporosis.

The Other Side of Exercise

Unless you're a policewoman, construction worker, gym teacher, or carpenter, your normal daily activities won't make a big impact on your cardiovascular health, muscle strength and endurance, or flexibility, which are important for general health and fitness and disease prevention, says Maggie Greenwood-Robinson, Ph.D., a certified nutrition consultant in Newburgh, Indiana, and author of *Natural Weight Loss Miracles*.

Aerobic exercise such as jogging or brisk walking for 30 minutes or more increases your body's ability to process and utilize oxygen. It keeps your heart and lungs healthy, and it can help prevent diabetes, high blood pressure, and certain types of cancers, says Janet P. Wallace, Ph.D., professor of kinesiology and associate professor and director of adult fitness at Indiana University in Bloomington.

Weight training, on the other hand, is an anaerobic workout. Your body doesn't have the same oxygen needs as it does when performing an aerobic exercise. Lifting weights builds lean muscle tissue, keeps you strong, gives you more energy, and prevents bone loss—a major concern for women in their postmenopausal years.

Then, there are flexibility exercises such as yoga and stretching to keep your muscles, ligaments, and tendons limber and less susceptible to injury, says Tia Willows, assistant vice president of group exercise at Bally Total Fitness in Chicago.

Exercise of any type can make you feel really good physically and psychologically after a stressful day. "It allows you to set aside a moment for yourself to relax and unwind. And it's a time to socialize if you participate in an exercise class," says Willows. The effects of exercise may go even deeper than that. Some researchers have shown that it can actually relieve depression and anxiety.

Exercise can also make you look younger. After you exercise, your skin tone will take on a youthful glow because working up a sweat increases blood circulation, which supplies nourishment to your skin and gives you a healthier appearance, says Dr. Greenwood-Robinson.

How Much Exercise Do I Need?

Increasing the frequency of your workouts, even if you're already active, may help you lose weight. Add an hour or two of exercise to your regular routine each week. "On average, 2 hours of activity will burn about 1,000 calories a week. You must burn 3,500 calories to lose 1 pound of fat. So in 3½ weeks, you can knock off 1 pound through exercise," says Dr. Greenwood-Robinson.

"Working in up to 2 hours a week of exercise is a very good short-term goal that many people won't find intimidating. If you start by walking

WOMEN ASK WHY

Why is it so difficult to lose belly fat even when I do regular aerobic exercise and stomach crunches and follow a low-fat diet?

Losing fat around your middle depends on your body type and what kind of exercise program you're following. Women are usually shaped like an apple, a pear, or an hourglass. If you have an apple shape, it's because you have a greater tendency to store fat around your tummy. Pear shapes store more fat on their hips and thighs. If you're lucky enough to have an hourglass figure, you'll seem to have fat in all the right places.

For flatter abs, stomach crunches and regular aerobic exercise usually do the trick, but not always. Crunches are ideal for strengthening and defining your abdominal muscles, but they won't help banish belly fat. Aerobic exercise is wonderful because it burns overall body fat and can whittle your waist. But if the fat still isn't budging, you'll need to turn up the calorie-burning heat with some resistance training.

Another contributor to belly fat is the decline in the female hormone estrogen that begins in our thirties. Doctors don't know why less estrogen means more abdominal fat, but do they believe there's a connection.

So what's the solution? Exercise aerobically for at least 30 minutes on most days of the week and add about 60 minutes of resistance training per week. You can break it up into three 20-minute sessions or two 30-minute workouts. Do a series of exercises for your upper and lower body with dumbbells or weight machines. Continue to do stomach crunches. Just add a variety of ab exercises to get the best results.

Expert consulted
Catherine Brumley
Certified trainer and fitness director
Canyon Ranch Health Resort in the Berkshires
Lenox, Massachusetts

or jogging for 20 minutes a day three times a week, you can get fit. You'll become stronger, and you'll be ready to push yourself to do more," says Sherry L. Granader, a nutritionist, certified aerobics instructor, and author of *The Eat Right, Feel Good, Lose Weight, Have Fun Cookbook*.

If you happen to work in a big city and can walk briskly for 10 to 20 minutes to and from your office, you're probably getting all the aerobic exercise you need. In that case, set aside 2 to 3 hours a week for weight training and stretching exercises to round out your fitness program, says Willows.

You'll condition your muscles and make your body a more efficient fat-burning machine, adds Dr. Wallace.

Now that you know how far a little exercise can go, here are a number of activities experts say that you can do to make physical activity fun and exciting. Before starting any exercise plan, however, check with your doctor.

Spinning

You'll be glad to know that twirling around in circles like a top is not the workout we're talking about here. Spinning is an aerobic, high-intensity indoor cycling class. With upbeat music jamming in the background, an instructor takes you through a warmup, hill climbs, descents, intervals of fast and slow riding, and a cooldown at various speeds and resistances. Here's what it does for you.

Health benefits: Spinning conditions your cardiovascular system and tones the muscles in your thighs, calves, buttocks, and hips.

Calorie burn: Spinning burns 260 to 660 calories per hour, depending on your weight and how intensely you pedal.

REAL-LIFE SCENARIO

She Works with Her Husband Every Day, but He's the Only One Getting Thinner

When Andrea turned 40, she took a long, hard look at herself. The experience was enlightening. She was tired of being a travel agent. She was bored with her red hair, and she hated the extra 30 pounds she'd put on over the past 2 decades. So she enrolled in an evening journalism class at a local college, lightened her hair to blond, and took out a membership at a local health club.

Her husband, Tom, was proud of her. He liked the renewed interest and zest she was showing for life. And to support her efforts, he also joined the health club so he could exercise with her. Besides, he could stand to lose a few pounds himself. They began going to the club regularly, and in no time at all, the pounds started coming off—of Tom. He seemed to lose weight overnight, while Andrea struggled for every ounce. Now she's getting frustrated, and she's beginning to feel that she doesn't want to go with him to the gym anymore. What can she do?

The first thing Andrea should do is stop comparing herself with her husband. On average, men lose weight much faster than women because they have a greater amount of lean muscle mass. The more muscle you have, the more fat your body can burn while you're resting and exercising. In addition, women are more likely than men to skip meals when trying to slim down, which is a big weight loss no-no. Whenever you go for long periods without food, your metabolism slows dramatically, making it virtually im-

Convenience factor: Classes are held at various health clubs. You can buy your own stationary bike designed for spinning and work out in the comfort of your own home. But without the direction of a fitness trainer, you may not burn as many calories—or have as much fun. "It's the environment you're in that makes spinning such great exercise. The instructor pushes you, the music pushes you, and the people in the class push you," says Willows.

possible to lose weight. And, as a whole, women are less active than men.

Then, there's the fact that Andrea is 40 years old. She's beginning her menopausal years, which means that her growth hormone levels are steadily dropping. This natural physiological process, unfortunately, causes women to lose muscle and gain fat.

What Andrea needs to do is combine cardiovascular exercise with weight training. The cardio will boost her metabolism, and the weight training will help her build muscle, which will accelerate her weight loss.

The great benefit of cardiovascular exercise is what happens after you're finished: Your metabolic rate stays charged for another 12 to 18 hours.

After her cardio workout, Andrea should strength train, alternating upper and lower body exercises every other day. For instance, she can work her chest, arms, and back on Monday and her legs, hips, and butt on Tuesday. She should avoid exercising the same muscle groups two days in a row.

Andrea will notice a dramatic change in her weight by combining cardio and strength training. She'll be conditioning her body to burn fat more efficiently. The exercises will give her a sense of control, reduce her appetite and stress, and give her the body she desires.

Expert consulted
Jan McBarron, M.D.
Director of Georgia Bariatrics
Columbus, Georgia

How often should I do this? Two to three times a week.

Kick Boxing

The word may conjure up images of spindly martial arts champions waiting to knock out their opponents or visions of David Carradine demonstrating Kung Fu in the Old West. But at your local health club or YMCA, kick boxing is a non-contact cardiovascular workout that combines aerobic exercise with shadowboxing to whip you into ringside shape.

It involves a series of kicking, punching, and blocking movements against an imaginary opponent that are choreographed to high-energy music. Classes often go by the names Kwando, Cardio Kickboxing, Cardio Kicks, Boxercise, Tae-Bo, or just kickboxing. Depending on the club, you may wear boxing gloves or hand mitts, use actual punching bags, or combine the movements with step aerobics. Check out the fitness bonuses.

Health benefits: Kickboxing is a total-body cardiovascular workout that sculpts and tones your arms, back, hips, thighs, calves, and abs. It also fine-tunes your sense of balance and coordination.

Calorie burn: You can burn 680 or more calories in a 1-hour class.

Convenience factor: Kickboxing classes are given at various health and fitness clubs across the country. You can also buy or rent kickboxing videotapes and do the routines at home.

How often should I do this? Two to three times a week.

Bowling

Who would have thought that bowling is actually a good work out? Well, repeatedly lifting and hurling a 6- to 14-pound ball, not to mention all that legwork, can do quite a bit for your figure. See for yourself.

Health benefits: You'll tone your throwing arm, hand, and shoulder as you release the ball. You'll strengthen your thighs, butt, and lower back during your approach, knee bend, and finish position.

Calorie burn: Bowling burns 204 calories an hour. Intensity depends on the number of games

WOMEN ASK WHY

If I spend 7 hours eating and I hour a week exercising, can I really lose weight?

Weight loss doesn't occur by keeping track of the time you spend eating and exercising. You lose weight by taking in fewer calories and expending more energy with regular exercise. You have to create a calorie deficit if you're going to drop those pounds.

You can potentially lose a pound of fat in a week without exercise if you cut 500 calories a day from your diet for 7 days. But if you decrease your calories too much without increasing physical activity, your body will slow its metabolism and store fat. Exercise turns your body into a more efficient calorie-burning machine.

So the key to slimming down is to eat slightly fewer calories—no matter how much time you spend doing it—and get moving. In fact, the more exercise you do, the less you have to worry about calories. Devoting just I hour a week to fitness really isn't sufficient. You won't burn enough calories to lose weight, you'll run the risk of injuring yourself, and you won't meet the recommendations for achieving optimal cardiovascular health. And, by burning 250 to 500 calories a day through exercise, you could lose up to a pound of fat a week—without restricting food.

According to the American College of Sports Medicine, you should get at least 30 minutes of aerobic exercise such as brisk walking, jogging, or cycling at least three to five days a week. If you find it impossible to fit in 30 minutes, break it up. Exercise for I0 minutes at a time in the morning, afternoon, and evening. The bottom line: Physical activity is the best way to burn calories and boost your metabolism to melt away the fat.

Expert consulted
Maggie Greenwood-Robinson, Ph.D.
Certified nutrition consultant
Newburgh, Indiana
Author of Natural Weight Loss Miracles

you play and the number of people you bowl with. More people means longer time lapses between turns, while bowling alone or with just one or two others keeps you moving more consistently.

Convenience factor: You must go to a bowling alley to reap the benefits.

How often should I do this? Two hours twice a week.

Table Tennis

If you have a Ping-Pong table packed away in your basement or garage somewhere, take it out, dust it off, and call a friend. Hitting a small, lightweight ball back and forth across a table actually counts as a real workout. Here's why.

Health benefits: Table tennis strengthens your quadriceps, hamstrings, inner and outer thighs, and hips.

Calorie burn: You can burn 270 calories per hour of steady playing. The type of workout you get is directly related to the level of skill with which you and your partner play. If you really want to start incinerating some calories and improving your game, find a friend who will like to practice a minimum of three times a week for about an hour each time.

Some tables fold up on one side so that you can play by yourself against the upended tabletop-a handy option if you can't find someone else to play as regularly as you'd like.

Convenience factor: All you need is a Ping-Pong table, two paddles, some balls, and a place to play.

How often should I do this? Three or four days a week.

Strength Training

Strength training simply means using dumb-bells or weight machines or some other form of resistance to strengthen and tone muscles in your upper and lower body. It burns lots of calories, takes years off your appearance, prevents many diseases associated with aging, and is the secret behind many a lean and strong woman, says Dr. Greenwood-Robinson. Here's what it can do for you.

Health benefits: Lifting weights builds muscle. And the more muscle you have, the more calories you burn at rest. Weight lifting shapes and sculpts your body (don't worry, you won't end up looking like a body builder unless you spend several hours a day in the gym or take steroids), boosts your metabolism around the clock, and helps prevent bone loss. You can shed pounds faster and maintain your weight more easily. And daily activities such as carrying groceries from your car to your front door will never be a problem, says Granader.

Calorie burn: Strength training burns up to 400 calories an hour and builds more muscle tissue. With more body-firming muscle, you're burning more calories, even while doing absolutely nothing.

Convenience factor: You can strength train at the gym or in your own home. All you need are a couple pairs of dumbbells, a weight bench, and a barbell with weight plates. Make sure you have someone spot you when you're using very heavy weights and aren't sure if you'll be able to complete a full set.

How often should I do this? Three 45-minute sessions per week.

Walking

Everyone knows that walking is as simple as putting one foot in front of the other. But if you want to lose weight, you'll have to walk like a woman on a mission—and pump your arms. In other words, power walk. Here's what you can expect if you do it regularly.

Health benefits: Your body will burn more calories and fat throughout the day because of the boost in your metabolism. You'll firm up the muscles in your buttocks, thighs, calves, back, upper arms, shoulders, and abdomen. You'll condition your cardiovascular system; reduce stress, heart disease, and stroke risk; help prevent osteoporosis; and elevate your mood, says Rebecca Gorrell, director of movement therapy at Canyon Ranch Health Resort in Tucson.

Calorie burn: Walking burns 100 calories per mile. You can burn 350 to 450 calories an hour, depending on how fast you walk and whether you hike on flat or hilly terrain.

Convenience factor: You can walk anytime and anywhere. There's no equipment to buy and no health clubs to join. All you have to do is lace up your walking shoes and head out the door or hop on a treadmill.

How often should I do this? Thirty to 40 minutes four or five times a week. For weight loss, five times a week for 40 minutes a session is recommended, says Gorrell.

Step Aerobics

Choreographed to the beat of heart-pumping music, step aerobics are high-intensity, low-impact exercises that combine dance moves on and around an adjustable platform. The "step" exploded onto the fitness scene in the late 1980s

TOP TOPS TIP
The Early Bird Catches the Burn

TOPS member Deborah Maier, 31, of Prairie Home, Missouri, struggled with her weight all her life. As an emotional eater since childhood, she often stuffed herself with food whenever she felt scared, stressed, angry, bored, sad, or happy. As a result, she had piled about 370 pounds on her 6-foot frame. And that put her health and her quality of life in jeopardy.

To deal with her weight problem, Deborah took on three challenges: She started eating low-fat, nutritious foods. She dealt with her emotions. And she began a regular exercise program. In just 18 months, she lost 202 pounds and went from a size 28 to a size 8 dress. Her current weight is 163 pounds. While combining all three strategies helped Deborah lose weight, she says that it was her daily morning exercise routine and TOPS that really made the impact.

At 8:00 A.M., Deborah hits the gym, where she runs 3 to 5 miles a day on the treadmill. After that, she does a series of weight training exercises and 150 abdominal crunches.

"Your metabolism runs on a 24-hour cycle," she says. "It's faster during the day and slower at night. Morning exercise gives your metabolism a boost before you start your day. And it stays elevated. It's like getting the most calorie burn for your buck. Working out in the afternoon is okay, but your body doesn't burn as many calories in the next 24-hour period because you gave your metabolism that charge later in the day."

calories in an hour using a 6-inch-high step.

Convenience factor: You can go to your local YMCA or health club and participate in a class, or you can buy a step bench and various step videos in some sporting goods stores or catalogs and work out at home.

How often should I do this? Two to 4 days a week.

Jogging

Like walking, jogging is one of the most accessible—and enjoyable—aerobic activities. But that's where the similarities end. Jogging burns calories a lot faster than walking, and it's one of the quickest ways to achieve cardiovascular fitness. Here's how it can pay off for you.

Health benefits: You strengthen and tone your abs and the muscles in your buttocks, hips, thighs, and calves. You build endurance, and your metabolic rate stays supercharged hours after you've completed your workout, says Dr. Greenwood-Robinson.

Calorie burn: Jogging burns 102 calories per mile. Depending on how fast your run, you can burn at least 500 to 600 calories in one hour.

Convenience factor: Jogging is almost as easy to do as walking. There are no lessons to take. No schedules to follow. No complicated moves to learn. Just lace up your running shoes and go.

How often do I need to do this? You can jog 3 to 5 days a week for 20 minutes or more per session.

and hasn't lost its popularity yet, says Granader. Here's how this high-energy class can help you drop those pounds.

Health benefits: You'll tone and shape the muscles in your buttocks, hips, thighs, calves, and abs. The arm movements will sculpt your biceps, triceps, and shoulders.

Calorie burn: Depending on the intensity of your workout, you can burn around 600

Paperback Writer: Your Life Story

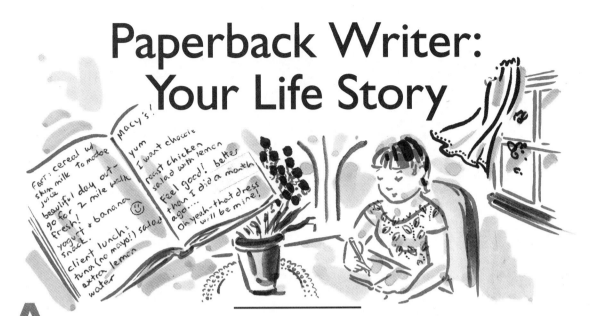

Anaïs Nin built her entire career around an opus of personal diaries, which she continued to write all of her life. She also remained impossibly thin all of her life. Coincidence?

Well, okay, maybe not, but keeping a diary—whether it's a personal journal, a food record, an exercise log, or a combination of all three—really can a be a helpful addition to your weight loss strategy.

"Given that dieting can be a challenge at best and a rather stressful experience at worst, it might be therapeutic to write down your deepest thoughts and feelings about your weight loss efforts," says Linda Cameron, Ph.D., senior lecturer in psychology at the University of Auckland, New Zealand, who has researched journaling extensively.

Through writing, you can also brainstorm coping strategies for stressful situations. If you're an emotional eater, you can use journaling instead of eating as a way to deal with feelings when you're upset. Finally, writing can serve as a way of monitoring your eating and activities. Keeping a food diary and/or exercise log can clue you in to bad habits that you may never have re-

alized you had. Then, as you begin to make changes in your lifestyle, you'll see proof of your progress toward a more active, thinner you.

Writing Down to the Bones

Many of us think that we eat less than we actually do. It's an easy mistake to make, nutritionists say, between the huge restaurant portions we've become accustomed to, our sometimes sketchy nutritional know-how, and our own absentmindedness about the calories in soft drinks, snacks, and other mindless munchies.

And we're not talking about a few pretzels and 50 calories. In one study, researchers found that some women miscalculated their daily caloric intake by an average of 621 calories a day—or more than half an angel food cake.

"The women in our study definitely underestimated their energy intake," says Mary Kretsch, R.D., Ph.D., a research nutrition scientist at the USDA Western Human Nutrition Center at the University of California, Davis.

A food diary can help. "When people start

watching what they're doing, they start to make changes," says Kerri Boutelle, Ph.D., a clinical psychologist at Children's Hospital in Minneapolis.

That's why food diaries represent a mainstay in many weight loss programs. Just the act of writing down what we're munching at meals and snacks makes us start making subtle changes in our diets. "It raises a woman's consciousness about what she's eating, which then allows her to make more healthful choices," explains Dr. Kretsch.

If you're ready to raise your consciousness with a food diary, here's how weight loss experts say you should do it.

Keep it portable. A 4-inch by 6-inch notebook represents the standard in many studies. You want a diary small enough to carry easily in your purse or pocket, yet with enough space to record everything from your portions to your emotions.

Track essentials. A handful of entries represent the backbone of your food diary. Each time you eat, record the time, whether it was a snack or a meal, the food and its preparation method (grilled chicken, steamed vegetables, a chocolate bar), serving size, calories, and fat grams. A pocket calorie counter can be an invaluable tool to help you keep track of the numbers.

But you can write about more than food in your food diary. Make room to write down your emotions and exercise. If, every time you eat, you jot down how you're feeling, you'll soon see if emotions are triggering your snack attacks. Reinforce your new active lifestyle by scribbling down exercise and activities, noting the calories burned.

WOMAN TO WOMAN

She Found Friends and Motivation through an Online Diary

When Tracey Peterson, 36, moved to Tuscaloosa, Alabama, 2 years ago, this native Californian was miserable. At 247 pounds, she could barely breathe, much less move, in the southern heat and humidity. Then, while watching Oprah one day, she realized that she could change her lifestyle to lose weight and become healthier and happier. The problem was that she didn't have the social support and encouragement that she wanted for her weight loss efforts—until she began an online diary. Here is her story.

When I started my diet, I knew absolutely no one—except for my husband—in Alabama. That was hard, because I didn't have friends to talk to or motivate me. Then a friend suggested I start an online diary.

When I discovered how motivating it could be to read other people's journals, I decided to write one of my own. I wanted to tell how it was to be overweight, including the emotions and physical strains that you experience. The more I wrote, the more people began to think that they had known me for years. The reaction I got was like a landslide. I was getting 100 e-mails a day from people all over the world. Women were finding hope and starting their diets because of my stories. Women who couldn't leave their houses because they were so heavy were now walking around the block. The more e-mail I got, the more motivating it was.

Rate your hunger. When was the last time you waited until you were truly hungry to eat? Can't remember? When we gain, lose, and regain the pounds over and over again, it may mean that we've started eating on autopilot and have forgotten what hunger feels like, suggests Gloria Kensinger, R.D., a registered dietician in Wheaton, Illinois. Rating your hunger from 0 to 5 (where 0 equals "starved" and 5 equals "stuffed") can reacquaint you with your body's hunger signals.

I've always been an open person, and I talk about everything in the diary, from physical problems to embarrassing moments. I felt that I owed it to people to talk about what we were all going through at different times. E-mails would pour in, all saying, "I thought I was the only one." I've also written about how depressed I felt when the weight wasn't coming off fast enough. You think your efforts aren't doing any good, and you just want to give up. Then the e-mails would arrive: "You can't give up; you're who I come to for motivation" or "Whenever I feel bad, I log on to your site for an inspirational quote." It keeps you going.

I definitely feel less isolated now. I've started getting e-mails from women in my town, and we're planning on meeting monthly for a walk or hike or just to talk with new friends.

Personally, writing helps you work through the bad times. Putting your feelings and thoughts down on paper—or on screen—releases what's built up inside. Afterward, you can read it and see where you need to make changes. When I first moved to Alabama, I had trouble breathing in the heat and humidity. I could barely go up and down the stairs. My knees hurt. My back hurt. But after a year of moving and breathing normally, I'd forgotten those problems—until I reread my journal. I'm grateful that I kept the diary because it reminds me of how I've grown.

Follow food groups. Trying to eat more whole grains? Fresh fruits? Green leafy veggies? Write your food group goal—for example, "five servings of fruits and vegetables"—in your food diary for every day. Then, track your progress: Make a check mark next to your goal each time you snack on carrots or choose fruit for dessert.

Time yourself. You also may want to record the minutes that you spend eating. Perhaps you're nibbling on the run more frequently than you realize or, even when you do sit down to eat, you're finished with your meal in 15 minutes or less. When you learn to eat more leisurely, you'll not only enjoy your food more but you'll also have the opportunity to stop eating when you feel full instead of when it's too late.

Record meals promptly. Don't wait until the day's end to write down what you had for breakfast. Who can remember 15 hours later how many ounces of orange juice she drank at 7 A.M.? Instead, jot down the details ("Breakfast: 4 ounces orange juice, one sesame seed bagel with 1 tablespoon cream cheese") immediately after you eat. You'll spend less time on the diary, because you won't be wracking your brain trying to recall what you ate hours ago, and your entries will be more accurate.

Work with a professional. If you're diligent about your food diary, you'll soon have pages of data about your eating habits. But you need more than information to make changes in your lifestyle; you need insight. Here's where a nutritionist can help. After looking at your entries, she can translate your food choices into nutrient intake, food groups, and more so that you can see the trends in your own eating patterns and ensure that you're getting the vitamins and minerals you need. "You need some way to evaluate where you are so that you can reach your health and nutrition goals," Dr. Kretsch says.

Look for patterns. Do you always eat dinner in front of the TV? Do you reach for chocolate ice cream when you're depressed? Do you overeat on the weekends while you're out with friends? Food diaries can help you uncover

TOP TOPS TIP

Embroidery Kept Her Busy

As a military bride living in rural Japan in 1970, TOPS member Beverly Enos needed a hobby that would occupy lots of time—and cake-decorating wasn't what her figure needed. She discovered bunka shishu, a form of Japanese embroidery. Stitched with silk or rayon threads, the wall hangings typically measure 16-by-20 inches or more and resemble delicate paintings. Now 50, Beverly owns her own bunka shishu gallery, Purple Dragon Arts, in Georgetown, Massachusetts, and credits the fine decorative art with helping her permanently lose 70 pounds.

"When I was in Japan, there was very little to do. There was no television. No radio. No paved roads. My husband was working rotating shifts, so I was alone for hours on end. I needed something to do that would take up long spans of time and not damage my body or my life. Then a neighbor taught me bunka shishu. You can't eat and stitch at the same time!"

You may not live in rural Japan, but you can still use needlework as a weight loss helper. Try cross-stitch embroidery, needlepoint, crocheting, knitting—anything that keeps your hands busy and your mind off food.

the situations that can undermine your weight loss. Once you know your high-risk situations, you can develop coping strategies.

Be honest. "People sometimes think, 'Oh, I'm going to see a dietitian—I better make this look good,'" says Julie Swanson, R.D., a clinical dietitian at Hennepin County Medical Center in Minneapolis. But fudging your food diary won't make the weight disappear; it'll just make it harder for your dietitian to spot problems or offer useful support in your efforts toward a thinner you.

Watch out for burnout. "You can't continue keeping a food diary indefinitely because

there's a fatigue factor," Dr. Kretsch says. Once you've discovered the hidden calories and eating triggers in your life and you've replaced them with healthier habits, you can probably take a break from recording every bite that you take. If you hit a weight loss plateau, though, grab your notebook and start writing; it will help you refocus on your goals and uncover the source of your weight loss standstill.

Be kind to yourself. You want your food diary to be accurate, but there's no need to be a perfectionist. "If you tend to be compulsive about eating or counting calories, a food diary can be a negative thing," Swanson cautions. "If keeping a food record is taking away from your goals by making you feel bad, put it away or use it as an occasional spot check to see how you're doing."

Dear Diary

As you can see, a food diary can serve as an invaluable tool in your weight loss efforts by helping you develop healthier eating habits. But, as we all know from past diets, successful weight loss involves more than counting calories and watching fat grams. We've done that; yet the scale keeps creeping back up. Perhaps the problem isn't our eating habits, but our "feeling" habits.

"Women often eat in a misguided effort to cope with stress," says Simone Ravicz, Ph.D., a licensed clinical psychologist in Pacific Palisades, California, and author of *High on Stress.*

Journaling represents a better way to deal with the stress in your life. Studies have shown that writing about stressful events can boost your immune system, reduce doctor visits, and even lessen the symptoms of chronic diseases such as asthma or rheumatoid arthritis. If journaling can benefit your physical health in such unexpected ways, imagine what it can do for your emotional health and, by extension, your weight loss.

"Writing about the stressful aspects of your life can help you resolve issues and, perhaps in the long run, reduce emotional distress, which is often a trigger for eating 'comfort' foods or overindulging," Dr. Cameron says. "People tend to go off diets when they're stressed." Or upset. Or angry. Or sad. Whatever you're feeling, a journal provides a safe place to vent and release those feelings before the emotional maelstrom drives you to seek comfort in food.

Journaling also provides a way to gain insight and understanding about the issues that you're facing as you lose weight. Perhaps your closest friend has been surprisingly unsupportive of your plans; maybe you're angry at yourself for not shedding pounds faster. Through writing, you can get some perspective on these emotional events. "Putting your feelings and thoughts into words helps you make sense of the experience," Dr. Cameron says. "You're also more able to identify potential coping strategies."

Journaling can be especially beneficial if you suspect that you're an emotional eater. If your food diary shows that you tend to overeat after

GUILT-FREE PLEASURE

These Are Not Your Mother's Romance Novels

Whether it's a chilly winter day or a lazy summer afternoon, there's nothing more delicious than curling up with a juicy read. Tucked away in a comfy chair, we quickly become engrossed in the latest bestseller—and completely forget about the leftover chocolate cake on the counter. But even the most avid readers tire of their usual literary mix.

Maybe it's time for a romance novel. If you've vowed that you'd never read one of those "bodice rippers," perhaps it's time to reconsider. Today's romance novels feature more diverse characters, plots, and styles than they used to. You'll find heroines who are doctors, lawyers, and single mothers—not just the traditional simpering servant girls you may remember from your mother's paperbacks.

"Just as women's lives have changed since the 1950s, so, too, have the story lines and characters in romance," says Rosemary Johnson-Kurek, Ph.D., an instructor at the University of Toledo in Ohio and co-editor of *Romantic Conventions*. "Any type of fiction can also be a romance."

Interested in a story with African-American characters? Try Shirley Hailstock or Beverly Jenkins. Have your children gotten you hooked on the *The X Files* with its spooky paranormal plots? Look for Maggie Shayne, whose books feature fantasy elements such as time travel and ghosts. Do you enjoy reading steamy love scenes? Katharine Kincaid is known for her sensual books. Are you a closet fan of the original "Thomas Crown Affair," with its handsome hero and art theft intrigue? Check out Elizabeth Lowell; her suspenseful adventures often involve jewels and other treasures.

"There's almost anything your heart desires," says Dr. Johnson-Kurek, who enjoys the requisite happy endings. "And there's nothing depressing about them."

a fight with your teenager or an outing with your mother, ask yourself why in your personal journal. "With journaling, you get direct insight into what's triggering the emotion and the ensuing cycle," Dr. Ravicz says. Once you know the trigger, you can stop the cycle.

If you're ready to start scribbling, here's what journaling experts recommend.

Take 20. No time to keep a diary? Think again. Writing for as little time as 20 minutes can improve your mood and health.

Write regularly. If you're dealing with a particularly traumatic experience, you may want to continue writing about it over a period of 3 to 5 days to allow yourself to work through your different emotions.

Tackle tough topics. To truly benefit from putting pen to paper, you must be willing to write about difficult issues. Rambling about superficial topics simply won't provide the same health advantages.

Be prepared. If you eat in response to stress, carry a notebook with you so that you can write instead of nibble when things get tense. "Writing isn't going to alleviate your hunger pangs, but it may help reduce impulse eating triggered by feelings of being unable to cope with stressful situations," Dr. Cameron says.

Don't try to distract yourself. If you're obsessing about food, don't try to divert your mind from food by writing about another topic; it will only make you more likely to run to the refrigerator. Focus on your thoughts and feelings about food instead. Why is it so important for you to eat right now? What does eating mean to you? How can you handle this situation?

Brainstorm solutions. While the Pollyannas of the world can scribble happily away, the pessimists among us need a little more structure to benefit from journaling. After you write about a problem, keep yourself from lapsing into negativity by spending 5 minutes thinking about new ways to approach the upsetting situation.

Say you're upset at a friend's disparaging comments about your weight. How can you handle this situation now and in the future? Jot down whatever ideas come to mind after you finish venting in your diary. You could take a walk, exercising away your anger rather than drowning it in a bowl of ice cream. Perhaps you could speak to her privately about her unkind words, telling her how hurt you felt and asking her to be more supportive. Maybe you could limit your outings with her—or stop them altogether until she begins acting like the friend you had thought she was.

The Art of Snacking: Eating Your Way to a Slimmer You

To anyone trying to lose weight, snack foods can seem like little devils, luring you toward disaster.

So at the grocery store, we zoom past the tortilla chips. At the movie theater, we dodge the oversize candy bars and skip over the buckets of buttered popcorn. And at our annual office parties, we run from the layer cakes, hop around the cookies, and head for the nearest exit at the sight of those luscious brownies.

But as often as we say no to temptation, the struggle never gets any easier. "The problem is that snacking is woven in to the very fabric of our culture," says Joan Salge Blake, R.D., a registered dietitian and adjunct clinical professor of nutrition at Boston University. "Many of our social activities center around food, whether it's a coffee break, a sporting event, or a meeting."

"Just turn on the television or flip through a magazine, and all you see are images of food. This appears to play a large role in women's snacking habits," says Ashini Shah, R.D., a registered dietitian at the Obesity Consultation Center at the New England Medical Center in Boston.

Yet, despite all the reminders of food that are thrown in our path each day, there's enormous pressure on women to look as shapely as Fran Drescher and as thin as Heather Locklear. Talk about a contradiction. "Women can be very weight-conscious, so they feel like they can't eat all those delicious snacks that they see out there. The situation definitely creates a big conflict," says Susan Olson, Ph.D., a clinical psychologist and weight management specialist in Seattle.

So how can we make our lives easier in the constant struggle to resist all those beckoning goodies? Easy. Give in.

Making an Angel out of the Snack Devil

Yes, of course, eating too many Hershey Bars and Twinkies (or any excess calories, for that matter) between meals can feed into gaining a dress size. But contrary to what many women believe, snacking can actually be a healthy and nutritious addition to any weight loss meal plan.

"The trick is to prepare in advance what

WOMEN ASK WHY

Why am I so hungry in the morning when I just had a large meal the night before?

Common sense tells us that it's because we haven't eaten in several hours. But the answer isn't that simple.

As part of the normal digestion process, your stomach produces acid after every meal. And the more food you eat, the more acid it makes.

If you overate at dinner, the extra acid remains in your tummy all night, along with the gastric juices that it normally creates after going without food for 8 to 9 hours. The end result is stomach acid overload, which can cause loud hunger pangs and a voracious appetite the next morning.

Your hunger also may be caused by fluctuating blood sugar levels. Whenever you overeat, your pancreas pumps out massive amounts of insulin—the hormone responsible for getting glucose, or sugar, into your cells so that it can be used as energy. If your cells reject the glucose (which is common in people who are overweight), your pancreas will dump out even more insulin to try to get the job done. Meanwhile, excess insulin and glucose are floating around in your bloodstream. Research shows that insulin does two things: It stimulates your appetite, and it produces body fat.

So how do you break this vicious cycle? Drink at least 4 ounces of water and take a chewable antacid such as Tums before you hit the sack. This will greatly reduce stomach acid. Read package directions for the correct dosage.

To level your blood sugar, eat a breakfast high in protein first thing in the morning—before you drink that cup of coffee. Oatmeal, yogurt, cottage cheese, eggs, and protein drinks made with soy milk are all good choices. If you drink coffee before you eat, your stomach will churn out that acid again. And that's what you want to avoid.

Expert consulted
Jan McBarron, M.D.
Director, Georgia Bariatrics
Columbus, Georgia

snacks you're going to eat. Have yogurt, fresh cut vegetables, and chopped fruit on hand so that you can dig right in when you're hungry," says Blake.

Second, make your snacks an extension to all your meals. If you plan to eat a bowl of cereal and some fruit for breakfast but can't finish it all, save your fruit for a mid-morning snack. If you buy a sandwich, soup, and a salad for lunch, eat your salad a couple of hours later. "It's a strategy that allows you to sneak in the fruits and vegetables that you didn't eat during your meals. And it keeps you from eating the higher-calorie stuff," Blake says.

But if you must have something sinfully sweet, buy chocolate bars and cookies in single-serving-size packages only. That way, you won't devour a whole box or bag, says Blake. "You'll be shocked to discover how satisfied you are with eating less."

Here's another snacking bonus: Healthy, planned snacking can prevent you from piling too much food on your plate for lunch and dinner. And that translates into fewer calories consumed.

Taming Those Midnight Temptations

While snacking has many advantages, it also has its disadvantages—especially if you're used to eating rocky road ice cream during episodes of late-night talk shows.

Why? Because at night, your body burns far fewer calories than it does during the day, which means that calories from what you eat after the sun goes down will likely show up as fat on your hips, butt, and thighs, says Audrey Cross, Ph.D., nutrition professor at the Institute of Human Nutrition at Columbia University in New York City. Here's how you can break the late-night-nibbling habit.

Stop skipping. The biggest error you can make if you want to lose weight is to skip breakfast and lunch and save your appetite for dinner. You'll be so hungry that not only will you eat a large dinner but you may also not stop eating for several hours afterward, warns Shah. And here's the real kicker: Because you'll be making up for lost meals, you'll consume the same number of calories—or more—in one sitting as you would normally eat throughout an entire day, she says.

Another drawback is that missing meals can drastically slow down your metabolism (the rate at which you burn fat and calories), says Maria Simonson, Ph.D., Sc.D., director of the health, weight, and stress clinic at Johns Hopkins Medical Institutions in Baltimore.

Fill 'er up. If you're not skipping meals but are still raiding the fridge at night, you're probably either not eating enough during the day or eating for reasons other than hunger, says Blake. "Women think that if they don't eat much during the day and eat a substantial dinner,

WOMEN ASK WHY

Why can I go without food all day at work and not be hungry but become ravenous when I get home?

When you're at work, your mind is focused on deadlines, meetings, phone calls, and other tasks. So food is the last thing you think about, especially if you're trying to drop a few pounds. Also, you may not feel hungry because you don't work around food. You don't see it or smell it, so you're not tempted to eat it.

You're starving by the time you get home for the obvious reason: You haven't eaten all day. But there's more to this story than meets the eye.

Women who have a habit of skipping breakfast and lunch feel deprived and even go so far as to make mental IOUs to themselves, saying, "Well, I missed two meals, but when I get home, I'm going to make up for it."

What's more, the moment the workday ends, your mind starts to relax, and the reality that you're hungry starts to sink in. When that happens, your body starts producing excessive amounts of stomach acid because you haven't eaten all day, and that makes you feel even hungrier.

While all this is going on, you're thinking about the comforts of home, which for many women means a time in their childhood when Mom fixed them a snack whenever they returned from school.

So the moment you step foot into the house, you and your appetite are totally out of control.

The solution? Eat breakfast and lunch and two healthy snacks to get you through your day. Keep apples, bananas, pears, pretzels, or saltine crackers in your car or at work. And before you head home, drink a large glass of water to dilute stomach acid. You'll take the edge off your hunger, and you'll be a lot less likely to raid the refrigerator.

Expert consulted
Jan McBarron, M.D.
Director, Georgia Bariatrics
Columbus, Georgia

they'll lose weight. But most often, that only leads to overeating," says Shah.

The solution? Eat breakfast, lunch, a snack, and then dinner. That way, you won't feel like devouring two bags of potato chips when that Lifetime movie you've been dying to see comes on, says Dr. Cross.

Break a sweat. Walk, jog, weight train, or participate in a team sport such as softball, soccer, or volleyball. Why? Because physical activity relieves stress and builds self-esteem and, as a result, you may be more inclined to eat healthier, says Shah. Accumulating 20 to 30 minutes of exercise daily could help curb appetite and munching.

The Top 20 Weight Loss Snacks

The smart way to graze is to choose lower-fat, fiber-rich, nutritious foods and to eat no more than the recommended serving size, says Kitty Gurkin Rosati, R.D., a licensed dietitian/nutritionist, nutrition director of the Rice Diet Program at Duke University in Durham, North Carolina, and author of *Heal Your Heart*.

Here's a list of the top 20 figure-friendly snacks that can fit into any woman's weight loss plan.

1. Freeze your fruit. Pluck some freshly washed grapes from a stem, arrange them on a small cookie sheet, and place them in the freezer. Once frozen, remove the grapes from the cookie sheet and enjoy. Store any remaining grapes in a zipper-top freezer bag and return to the freezer for up to 2 months. Serving size: ½

REAL-LIFE SCENARIO
She Sabotages Her Health with Late-Night Snacks

Lindsey, 42, makes a promise to herself every morning: Today, she will cut down her calories, do her daily exercise, and eat nothing in the evening after dinner. Why? She wants to lose 35 pounds. So every day, she pedals for 20 minutes on her stationary bike, grabs a cup of coffee for breakfast, and eats cottage cheese for lunch. For dinner, she has a full-course meal, including potatoes or pasta, a green vegetable, and chicken or fish. But around 10 P.M., she begins to feel famished. She struggles with her conscience ("Remember your promise, Lindsey"), but corn chips beckon from the pantry. She tells herself that she'll eat one serving: just 9 chips. But one serving turns into two, which can sometimes turn into an entire bag. Afterward, she feels nothing but guilt and self-loathing. And she has yet to lose her first ounce. How can she help herself?

Lindsey is getting off to a good start by beginning each day with 20 minutes of fat-burning aerobic exercise. But in order to reach her weight loss goals, she has to change her eating habits. Like many women battling to lose weight, Lindsey is skipping breakfast, skimping on lunch, and saving her appetite for dinner.

Whenever you miss meals, you deprive yourself of all the important vitamins and minerals that your body needs. You can end up feeling hungry and cheated, and you set yourself up for unhealthy, impulsive snacking later on in the day. The reason why Lindsey is famished shortly after her dinner is because she probably doesn't eat enough to compensate for the breakfast and lunch that she skips earlier.

cup grapes; 60 calories, 0 gram fat. Another tip: Peel a banana, cover it in plastic wrap, and place in a zipper-top freezer bag. Freeze and eat. Serving size: 1 medium banana; 105 calories, 0 gram fat.

2. Roast your veggies. Preheat your oven to 350°F. Spray a baking pan with olive oil. Chop

As a result, she turns those corn chips into a full-course meal.

To drop those 35 pounds, Lindsey needs to start eating breakfast and lunch on a daily basis. Pumping fuel into her body early in the day can help prevent her from bingeing on chips and other fattening fare late at night. Her breakfast can consist of cereal, fat-free milk, and fruit; half of a whole grain bagel with melted low-fat cheese on top; cottage cheese, fruit, and an English muffin with jelly; or a cup of yogurt, a banana, and a low-fat whole grain muffin.

For lunch, she can have a chicken, roast beef, or tuna sandwich; a small salad topped with fresh vegetables, beans, and low-fat dressing; or a bowl of vegetable soup, a piece of fruit, and some yogurt. If that's too much to eat in one sitting, she can save the fruit and yogurt for a mid-afternoon snack. She won't be as hungry, and she'll more than likely eat smaller portions at dinner.

If Lindsey still feels hungry a couple of hours later, she should identify the nutritious foods that she didn't get a chance to eat earlier. For instance, if she didn't meet her daily requirements for fruits and vegetables, that's what she should eat. If she didn't get enough dairy, she should have yogurt. If she still wants a snack after she has met her needs, she can choose a small serving of whatever she wants. But by that time, her snack will remain a snack. It won't turn into a meal.

Expert consulted
Joan Salge Blake, R.D.
Registered dietitian
Adjunct clinical professor of nutrition
Boston University

some eggplant, bell peppers, onions, sweet potatoes, asparagus, mushrooms, and garlic and place them on the pan. Roast them for 15 minutes, turn them over, and cook for another 15 minutes, or until the vegetables are browned. Serving size: ½ cup; 25 to 100 calories, less than 1 gram fat. (Calorie and fat counts will be dependent on the amount of oil and type and portion of vegetables used.)

3. Make your own chips. You'll need 24 fat-free, salt-free tortillas, garlic powder, cumin, chili powder, and olive oil spray. Preheat oven to 350°F. Lightly coat the baking sheet with olive oil spray. Cut each tortilla into eight equal pieces and spread them over the baking sheet. Bake for 10 minutes, or until the chips curl and turn slightly brown. Remove from oven and spray lightly with cooking spray. Sprinkle with the seasonings suggested, or try your own combinations to find your favorite. Serving size: 8 chips; 67 calories, 1 to 2 grams fat.

4. Whip up a dip. Pour one 16-ounce can of no-salt, low-fat refried beans and 6 ounces of no-salt salsa into a bowl. Blend in the juice of one lime, 2 tablespoons chopped fresh cilantro, and some minced fresh jalapeño chile peppers to taste (wear plastic gloves when handling). Mix well. Serving size: ½ cup; 134 calories, 2 grams fat. Beware of pickled jalapeños; they're loaded with sodium. This dip goes great with the chips above.

Note: No-salt refried beans can be a little difficult to find, but they're definitely worth the effort.

5. Savor some cereal bars. The low-fat versions of these fruit-filled snacks come in a wide variety of flavors. Serving size: 1 bar; 130 calories, 3 grams fat.

6. Blaze your own trail mix. Mix together three of your favorite low-fat, whole grain cereals in a large bowl. Look for bran or whole wheat cereals that contain at least 2 to 3 grams of fiber and less than 8 grams of sugar per serving.

TOP TOPS TIP

Planned Snacking Made Her Weight-Loss Program Work

A diet consisting of hamburgers, French fries, fried chicken, and high-fat snacks caused former substitute teacher Fran Condo Drozdz of Litchfield, Arizona, to pile on an unhealthy 30 pounds that she struggled to lose for years. To get rid of her fat, she popped diet pills and tried every fad diet imaginable. The problem was that whenever she lost some weight, she regained it quickly—until she found a more permanent solution: regular exercise, low-fat meals, and lots of planned snacking.

She hasn't looked back since. Fran, 56, dropped those 30 pounds 17 years ago, and not one of them has returned. Her 20-year membership with TOPS and her plum position as their health and fitness spokesperson/ambassador has played a key role in her success. She offers women advice on how to keep weight off for good, and she even gives away these weight loss snacking secrets.

Carry a cooler. Pack a small plastic cooler with you wherever you go, in case you get hungry. Fill it with bagels, jam, apples, bananas, yogurt, and low-fat cheese sticks. You'll avoid stopping at fast-food restaurants, convenience stores, and vending machines.

Prepack your snacks. Select 10 of your favorite low-fat snacks and put 100 calories worth of each in separate plastic bags. Got the munchies? Just grab a bag and chow down. You'll always know exactly how much you're eating, and you'll never feel deprived. Some of Fran's bagged favorites include pretzels, Fig Newtons, low-fat popcorn, flavored rice cakes, low-fat trail mix, and prunes.

cles are terrific, too. Serving size: 1 bar; 40 to 100 calories, 0 to 1.5 grams fat.

8. Scoop some pudding. Try the low-fat and fat-free varieties in single-serving containers, available in assorted flavors. Serving size: 1 container (3.5 ounces); 100 calories, 0 gram fat. Also try fat-free instant pudding mix. Serving size: ½ cup; 90 calories, 0 gram fat.

9. Pack pretzels. Available in their regular, low-fat and fat-free varieties. Serving size: 1 ounce; 100 calories, 0 gram fat. Dip them in mustard or barbecue sauce.

10. Pop some corn. Choose the low-calorie, fat-free microwave varieties. Eat as many as 6 cups, and you'll still be under 150 calories. Serving size: 1 cup; 15 calories, 0 gram fat. Another option: Air-pop your own popcorn. Then lightly spray the popcorn with olive oil and sprinkle it with chili powder, garlic powder, onion powder, pepper, cinnamon, or fat-free Parmesan cheese.

11. Devour some yogurt. Choose low-fat or fat-free varieties. Average serving size: 6 to 8 ounces. Low-fat: 170 to 220 calories, 2 to 3.5 grams fat. Fat-free: 120 calories, 0 gram fat.

12. Feast on figs. Fat-free fig bars are available in cranberry, raspberry, and strawberry flavors. Serving size: 2 cookies; 100 calories, 0 gram fat.

13. Enjoy some veggies. Buy some precut, bagged, fresh vegetables that include broccoli, carrots, and cauliflower. Dip them in your favorite creamy, fat-free salad dressing. Serving size (veggies): ½ cup; 35 calories, 0 gram fat.

Serving size: 1 cup; approximately 100 calories, 1.5 grams fat.

7. Scream for ice cream. Low-fat, low-calorie ice cream, fat-free frozen yogurt, and sorbet are available in decadent flavors. Serving size: ½ cup; 130 calories, 0 to 5 grams fat. Frozen yogurt and fruit juice Popsi-

TOP 10 SUBSTITUTES

Looking for scrumptious low-calorie snacks that won't make you feel deprived? Here's a list of the top 10 snack alternatives to the fattening treats that will satisfy your sweet tooth—and help shrink your waistline.

Eat this . . .	Instead of this . . .
1. ½ cup Häagen-Dazs fat-free frozen yogurt Vanilla raspberry: 130 calories, 0 g fat Chocolate sorbet: 120 calories, 0 g fat	½ cup Häagen-Dazs ice cream Vanilla: 270 calories, 18 g fat Chocolate: 270 calories, 18 g fat
2. ½ cup Edy's Coffee Fudge Sundae fat-free frozen yogurt: 100 calories, 0 g fat	Edy's Grand Ice Cream Double Fudge Brownie: 170 calories, 9 g fat
3. 1 Weight Watchers Smart Ones Mocha Java Bar: 80 calories, 1.5 g fat	1 Dove Bar: 260 calories, 17 g fat
4. 4 oz Jell-O Fat-Free Pudding Snacks: 100 calories, 0 g fat	4 oz Jell-O Pudding Snacks: 159 calories, 5.1 g fat
5. 1 oz (15 chips) Pringles fat-free potato chips: 70 calories, 0 g fat	1 oz (14 chips) Pringles regular potato chips: 160 calories, 10 g fat
6. 1 package (6 sandwiches) Nabisco Cheese Crackers with Cheddar Cheese: 200 calories, 11 g fat	38 Snackwell's Zesty Cheese Snack Crackers: 130 calories, 3 g fat
7. 1 oz (6 chips) Tostitos WOW Restaurant-style: 90 calories, 1 g fat*	1oz. (7 chips) Tostitos Restaurant-style: 140 calories, 6 g fat
8. 1 oz (about 18 chips) Guiltless Gourmet Baked Organic Tortilla Chips (red corn, chili lime, blue corn, black bean): 110 calories, 2 g fat	1 oz (12 chips) Doritos Tortilla Chips (nacho cheese, cool ranch, spicy nacho, smoky red BBQ, Baja picante): 140 calories, 7 g fat
9. 1 cup popped Orville Redenbacher's 94% Fat-free Butter Smart Pop: 15 calories, 0 g fat	1 cup popped Orville Redenbacher's Movie Theatre Butter Popcorn: 40 calories, 3.5 g fat
10. 7 Quaker Crispy Mini Caramel Corn Cakes: 60 calories, 0 g fat	⅔ cup Crunch 'n' Munch Buttery Toffee Popcorn with Peanuts: 150 calories, 6 g fat

*Contains Olestra, which may cause abdominal cramping and loose stools. Olestra inhibits the absorption of some vitamins and other nutrients.

Serving size (dressing): 2 tablespoons; 35 to 50 calories, 0 gram fat.

14. Grab a bagel. It will fill you up and boost your energy. Serving size: ½ bagel; 105 calories, 0 gram fat. Slathering it with 1 tablespoon jelly adds 40 to 50 calories, 0 gram fat; 2 tablespoons fat-free cream cheese adds 30 calories, 0 gram fat.

15. Palm some fruit. Apples, peaches, pears, and oranges are great for grab-and-go snacks. Serving size: 1 piece; 100 calories or less, 0 to 0.7 gram fat.

16. Jiggle some gelatin. Naturally fat-free and available in several flavors. Serving size: $\frac{1}{2}$ cup; 80 calories, 0 gram fat. There's also sugar-free. Serving size: $\frac{1}{2}$ cup; 10 calories, 0 gram fat.

17. Munch on rice cakes. Rice cakes come in many flavors. Serving size: 5 fat-free mini cakes; 50 calories, 0 gram fat.

18. Bake an apple. Core and peel the top third of a large (9 ounces) baking apple. Spoon 2 tablespoons low-fat granola, 1 tablespoon brown sugar, and a dash of ground cinnamon into the apple. Drizzle with 1 tablespoon caramel flavor sundae topping. Cover and microwave for 3 minutes, or until the apple is tender. Serving size: 1 apple; 245 calories, 3 grams fat.

19. Pass the taters. Slice an unpeeled, freshly scrubbed potato into thin wedges and place on a baking sheet spritzed with a cooking spray. Sprinkle the wedges with pepper and paprika and bake at 425° to 450°F for 15 minutes, or until done. Serving size: 1 potato with spices; about 230 calories, 0 gram fat.

20. Nosh on nachos. Preheat the oven to 325°F. Place 15 baked restaurant-size tortilla chips on a baking sheet lightly sprayed with a nonstick cooking oil. Top each chip with grated low-fat Cheddar cheese, fat-free bean dip, and salsa. Heat in the oven for 5 minutes, or until the cheese is melted and the dip and salsa are warm. Calories and fat will vary with the topping and chips used.

Home for the Holidays: Enjoying the Feast

Few things in life are as certain as this fact: You can't escape food during the holidays.

Glossy magazine covers display photographs of the perfect turkey, the ultimate gingerbread house, a Yule log cake. Department stores highlight their gourmet holiday goodies. Tins of baklava, chocolate-covered cherries, and tiny cakes arrive daily at the office. Each weekend brings an open house, a company party, a family celebration.

No wonder we gain a pound a week between Thanksgiving and New Year's. But it doesn't have to be that way. With a little seasonal savvy, we can make our way merrily through the holidays with our weight intact.

Take a Break

While the holidays may bring miracles, you shouldn't expect them weight-wise during the festive season.

"The holidays are problematic for everybody," says Kerri Boutelle, Ph.D., a clinical psychologist at Children's Hospital in Minneapolis. Seasonal obligations such as shopping or socializing disrupt our normal eating and exercise routines. If we're not traveling to be with family, we're frantically cooking and cleaning for our own holiday fetes. Not surprisingly, weight loss can become more difficult.

That's why many experts advise taking a "maintenance break" during the holidays. Instead of trying to shed pounds in the face of overwhelming temptation, focus on keeping your weight stable from Thanksgiving to New Year's. It sounds simple, but it's a significant accomplishment during the holiday season.

Such a break can benefit your physique and your psyche. Since weight loss often depresses your metabolism, a maintenance break "might give your body time to physically adapt to your new body size and allow your metabolic rate to adjust itself," says Josephine Connolly-Schoonen, R.D., clinical assistant professor of family medicine at the State University of New York in Stony Brook. "On the flip side, you'll reduce your own expectations."

By keeping your holiday weight goals realistic, you'll avoid the feelings of failure that often lead to bingeing, and you'll be more likely to stick to

WOMEN ASK WHY

Why do I crave only things that are bad for me and never things that are good?

Some researchers believe that women crave and consume foods such as chocolate because they contain essential nutrients or make women feel good. But others believe that the research tells a very different story: that women crave foods because of sensory, psychological, and behavioral factors. In other words, they crave foods that taste good, or foods that they associate with good things like love and holidays and special memories.

They also crave foods that they deprive themselves of. That's why we often crave high-fat or high-sugar foods instead of vegetables. But how do we know that it isn't some chemical in the food that makes us crave it?

At the University of Pennsylvania in Philadelphia, researchers studied chocolate cravers. They gave one group a chocolate bar and a second group all the chemicals in a chocolate bar, only in a capsule. The third group got white chocolate, which has no cocoa (and none of chocolate's chemical compounds). If chocolate contained substances that by their chemical nature would relieve cravings, then the capsule should have relieved people's cravings. It didn't. The only thing that relieved the cravings was the chocolate bar. That seems to say that there's something else that's important besides the chemicals.

Women make many judgments about cravings and foods; some foods are "bad" and some are "good." If a woman allows herself to eat foods that she has labeled as bad, then she feels guilt and shame. Some women are so hypersensitive about "bad" foods that any time they feel like eating that food, they think they're craving it. Relax a bit about your desire to eat foods that you may not feel are the absolute healthiest for you.

Expert consulted
Mindy S. Kurzer, Ph.D.
Associate professor, food science and nutrition
University of Minnesota
St. Paul

your weight loss plans as your successes build.

More Holiday Helpers

Whether you want to lose 5 pounds or 50, a handful of holiday hints will help you make it to January with your waistline intact. Here's a strategic sampler from weight loss experts around the country.

Maintain your routine. Don't skip your afternoon walk because you don't have time for your usual 30-minute loop. Do what you can, even if it's 10 minutes. "Half of what you're doing is preserving the habit of putting on your shoes and getting out the door," says Karen Kemper, Ph.D., associate professor in the department of public health science at Clemson University in South Carolina. "Once you lose a habit, it's hard to reestablish it." Come January 2, you'll have time to resume your regular route, and you'll have maintained the habit.

Keep that diary handy. Even if you don't keep a food journal at any other point during the year, now is the time. In one study, people who used a food diary religiously lost about $3/4$ pound a week, even during the holidays; the less diligent gained nearly a pound a week.

Bring in reinforcements. As helpful as a food diary can be, jotting down everything you nibble can get tedious. Friendly reminders can keep you motivated. Women and men who received phone calls, comic strips, and postcards from researchers reminding them about the importance of food diaries lost an average of 2 pounds during the holidays, while their counterparts, who did not get reminders, gained 2 pounds. "Anything you can do to remind yourself to keep your food diary helps, whether it's putting your diary where you can see it every day or leaving reminder notes for yourself around the house," Dr. Boutelle says.

Get ahead of the curve. If you've reached your goal weight, give yourself leeway by losing a few extra pounds prior to the holidays, advises Jan McBarron, M.D., director of Georgia Bariatrics, a medical center for overweight people in Columbus, Georgia. "Every fall, I drop 3 pounds before Thanksgiving. Between then and January 2, I can gain that 3 pounds back and be fine. It's not enough to notice, but it's enough to keep me where I need to be," says Dr. McBarron, who has lost 70 pounds and kept it off for more than 10 years.

Puttin' On the Ritz

In December, calendars fill quickly with social occasions: a neighbor's open house, a client's cocktail party, the company's annual dinnerdance. They're wonderful opportunities to dress up, mingle with friends, and taste a tableful of goodies. What's a holiday gathering without canapés and cocktails?

A chance to escape with my waistline intact, you may think.

Maybe so, but we don't have to forgo the mer-

rymaking because we're losing weight. We simply need to make smart choices about when and how to indulge when we're out and about. Here are some of the smartest choices that experts say you can make.

Don't skip meals to "save" calories. You'll arrive at the party ravenous and end up overindulging.

Forget the "new math." It's fine to eat a lighter lunch if you'll be attending an evening event; just don't give yourself too much credit for the calories you banked. "You may have saved a few hundred calories, but you didn't save 1,000," reminds Connolly-Schoonen. "People often give themselves permission to binge."

Spoil your appetite. A light snack an hour before a party will take the edge off your hunger and help you make better food choices. Try half a sandwich with a glass of fat-free or low-fat milk, a piece of fruit with cheese, or a small bowl of instant oatmeal.

Arrive late. The buffet doesn't look quite so appetizing once the partygoers start picking out the strawberries and spilling sauce on the rice.

Survey the table. By scanning the buffet before you fill your plate, you give yourself the power to craft a healthy, balanced meal that you'll enjoy, instead of worrying about leaving room for the unknown dishes at the table's end.

Go veggie. As always, your best picks will be the raw veggies. They're crunchy, filling, and low-fat—as long as you go easy on the dip.

Be careful of quick breads. Treats such as muffins and pumpkin and banana breads are higher in fat than yeast breads such as wheat or seven-grain.

Think plain. Lean proteins such as turkey, chicken, or fish—sans the fat-filled creamy sauces or breaded coatings—are healthy choices.

Go nuts. A *small* handful of nuts provides the fat (and it's the healthy kind, too!) you need to feel satisfied, especially if you're snacking on raw cauliflower and broccoli.

Skirt the buffet. If you're not standing 6 inches from the stuffed mushroom caps and those handy cocktail toothpicks, you won't keep nibbling on them.

REAL-LIFE SCENARIO
She Just Can't Bring Herself to Skimp On Holiday Meals

Valerie, 47, comes from a large, close-knit family, and she loves to see them as often as she can, especially during the holiday season, when they all bring their families over for a big holiday meal. Every family brings an entrée, a side dish, and a dessert. In the tradition of her family's roots, as dinner begins, she serves a full course of various ethnic foods. When that's finished, the table is cleared for a second complete meal of "American traditional food." Then come the pastries and fruits and nuts and cheeses. This year, however, she has been struggling very hard with weight loss, and she has been trying to eat only moderately sized healthy meals. She doesn't have the heart to foist her new diet on her family, but she knows that if they do the usual holiday meal, she won't be able to resist the feast. How can she help herself?

Valerie can help herself this holiday season in many ways.

First, to keep herself from feeling deprived, Valerie should sample everything that's appealing to her. Deprivation will only lead to more frustration.

Second, Valerie should remember that this happens only once a year. People often focus on what they eat from Thanksgiving to New Year's, but they'd be better off watching their diet and exercise habits the other 10½ months of the year. There are many temptations during the holiday season that people don't manage well. But they don't manage deprivation well, either.

Of course, her family could make changes in their cele-

Watch the wassail. Not only are you drinking the calories (68 in a 3½-ounce glass of white wine), you'll probably end up eating more, according to one study.

Mingle more than you munch. Focus on your friends and colleagues more than the food.

Get romantic. Still can't keep your paws off the buffet? "Hold your date's hand," suggests bration. Instead of each family bringing a full meal, they could each just bring their favorite dish. As a group, they could pick the "best of the best" from their ethnic and American meals, combining the winners in a single holiday feast.

Valerie could also make one change in each dish to cut down on fat and calories. Perhaps she could add flavor to the stuffing with chicken broth and avoid using butter. Maybe she could prepare pumpkin pie with fat-free evaporated milk rather than regular evaporated milk. These little savings add up.

She also could reconsider the desserts. Maybe there's a sweet treat on the table, such as lemon meringue pie, that she serves during the year. If a dish isn't truly special, maybe Valerie can remove it from the menu or simply forgo it herself. Valerie should save her calories for a small serving of the desserts that are most traditional and meaningful for her, such as the pecan or pumpkin pies that she eats just once a year, and savor every bite.

What we're really talking about is making some little changes in Valerie's family traditions. Those changes don't have to happen all at once. If this year, Aunt Tilly discovered that she has high cholesterol, Uncle Ned found out his blood pressure is too high, and Valerie is trying to lose weight, the family might just focus a little more on health. That doesn't mean the food won't be tasty. And they'll still honor those cherished family traditions.

Expert consulted
Melanie Polk, R.D.
Director of nutrition education
American Institute for Cancer Research
Washington, D.C.

brations. We're not only encountering tempting foods on the table but we're also face-to-face with the cooks themselves. "How do you deal with Grandma's pie *and* Grandma, especially when she starts saying, 'Oh, have another slice' or 'You really want a bigger piece'?" asks Judith S. Stern, R.D., Sc.D., professor of nutrition and internal medicine at the University of California, Davis. Just the thought of such an exchange makes us quail—and quickly justify the extra calories in the name of family harmony.

But unless we want to wake up New Year's morning with even more pounds to lose, we need to respond to such scenarios in healthier ways. "You have to chart your course ahead of time," Dr. Stern explains. "You have to be light about it, but you must be determined."

Here's a handful of strategies for sidestepping culinary pressures from family or friends this holiday season.

Confide in the hostess. If you're going to a friend or family member's house for a holiday meal, let her know your weight loss plans. "Tell her that you're watching your weight and to please not be insulted if you don't take large portions," Polk suggests. She'll be less likely to pressure you to eat more than you'd like.

Go potluck. Afraid you'll find nothing you can eat without guilt on your grandmother's groaning table? Provide a side dish that you know is low-cal. "You should be the one bringing the huge bowl of salad," Connolly-Schoonen says. Grandma will appreciate the help, and you'll have at least one healthy option to enjoy.

Melanie Polk, R.D., director of nutrition education at the American Institute for Cancer Research in Washington, D.C.

Facing the Family

As challenging as cocktail parties can be, they're child's play compared with family cele-

TOP TOPS TIP

A Thinner Thanksgiving Dinner

Jerilyn Tunell, 35, of Independence, Missouri, grew up in a southern family where lard was the shortening of choice. Those culinary calories added up. By the time Jerilyn was in her thirties, she weighed more than 350 pounds. So she began exploring healthier ways to prepare family favorites, even daring to modify (gasp!) traditional Thanksgiving dishes. The proof is in the fat-free pudding: Jerilyn and her husband have lost 350 pounds between the two of them. Here are her hints on cooking healthfully this Thanksgiving.

"You almost feel like, 'Oh, I can't change this recipe—the women in my family have cooked this dish this way for 40 years.' But you have to get past the emotions. Your grandmother in heaven isn't going to say, 'You terrible person. You used low-fat whipped topping on the pumpkin pie instead of whipped heavy cream!' She's going to look down and think you're taking care of yourself."

To create a healthier holiday meal, Jerilyn draws on a host of lower-fat alternatives. She uses applesauce instead of oil in banana bread. She replaces the butter in butterscotch yams with a fat-free butter substitute. She cooks the turkey in Reynolds cooking bags, which keeps the meat moist without basting. Her all-purpose substitute of choice? Chicken broth. She uses fat-free, no-salt chicken broth in everything from mashed potatoes to gravy.

Jerilyn admits that these alternatives can add dollars and cents to the holiday grocery bill, but just as it's okay to update Grandma's favorite biscuits, it's also okay to spend a few extra dollars on leaner meats or butter substitutes. "The battle is really in your head," the coordinator in charge of 140 TOPS chapters says. "You need to forgive yourself and say, 'I'm worth this. My health—my family's health—is worth buying quality ingredients for this recipe.'"

Of course, a healthy meal helps no one if everybody orders pizza in disgust. What did Jerilyn's family think of her first low-fat Thanksgiving feast? "They didn't know," she says. "They couldn't tell the difference."

Compliment the cook. If you're worried about offending your mother by eating less than a plateful of sweet potatoes, take a small portion of food and praise it effusively. "It goes farther than eating a huge amount and saying nothing," says Laurel J. Branen, R.D., Ph.D., associate professor of food and nutrition at the University of Idaho in Moscow.

Serve yourself. You can control what and how much goes on your dinner plate.

Taste your favorites. "If this is the only time of year where you get pumpkin pie, you don't want to give that up," Dr. Branen says. Just keep your portion size under control.

Don't clean your plate. If someone gives you more stuffing than you requested, don't finish it out of guilt. Dr. Branen says that her husband stopped her obsessive clean-plate club habit with one comment: "He said, 'It can go to waste in the garbage or it can go to "waist" in your body, but either way, it's going to waste.' He was right."

Get busy. What Thanksgiving chef could refuse an extra pair of hands after the meal is done? By offering to help with the postfeast cleanup, you'll take your mind off food, and no one will notice that you didn't request seconds of Aunt Edna's fruitcake.

Lie. When all else fails, tell your hostess that you're under the weather. "If you say that you're not feeling well, people understand and don't force extra food on you," Dr. Stern says.

What's Cooking?

If you're the chef this holiday season, you have a wonderful opportunity to make this year's feast a healthier one. Each Thanksgiving, the average American consumes an incredible 4,500 calories and 229 grams of fat—3,000 calories from the meal alone and 1,500 from pre- and postdinner snacking.

Of course, standing over the stove brings its own temptations.

Dr. Branen recalls one woman who swore that she didn't nibble while she cooked—until she tried wearing a surgical mask while she prepared a meal. "You get amnesia when you eat standing up," she says.

If you know you'll be cooking up a storm, experts suggest you try the following to keep your feasting—and tasting—under control.

Distract your tastebuds. You'll be less likely to nibble after you've freshened your breath by brushing your teeth, chewing gum, or sucking on a peppermint candy.

Stop tasting. "You've been making these holiday dishes for years," Connolly-Schoonen says with a laugh. "You probably know how to prepare them by now."

Spice things up. Instead of baking sweet potatoes with butter and marshmallows, try orange or pineapple juice with ginger, mace, and cinnamon.

Choose broth. You'll save fat and calories by substituting low-fat chicken broth for butter when preparing stuffing. Cook potatoes in broth

GUILT-FREE PLEASURE
Mistletoe

When we're trying to lose weight during the holidays, it can seem like every seasonal indulgence, from fruitcake to nuts, is off-limits.

Except for one.

Grandma's pumpkin pie can never compete with the calorie-free treat of kissing your honey under the mistletoe.

With its white berries and golden-green leaves, the plant has been helping people celebrate the seasons long before the first Christmas. The Druids, ancient Celtic priests, burned mistletoe at midsummer bonfires. Hundreds of years later, in 18th-century England, young men and women of different social classes would use the holiday decoration as an excuse to steal a kiss from someone they could only dream of the rest of the year.

The daring lovers had to act fast. Each bundle of greenery had only so many smooches.

"Each time the mistletoe was used, the couple had to remove a berry," explains Emma L. Powers, a historian with the Colonial Williamsburg Foundation in Virginia. "When the berries were gone, there were no more kisses."

By the way, those berries are poisonous, so if you decide to follow the same tradition, make sure you keep them away from the kids and pets.

to pump up the flavor, enabling you to skip the butter for mashing.

Bake smart. You can usually reduce sugar in a recipe by one-quarter without affecting the taste, says Stephanie Wilkins, a dietitian in Tuscaloosa, Alabama. She also suggests replacing butter or oil in baked goods with an equivalent amount of applesauce.

Start with soup. You'll feel full faster on fewer calories if you serve a broth-based soup as a first course.

Be inefficient. Dr. Stern clears her Thanksgiving table one dish at a time, making multiple trips between kitchen and dining room to keep her body moving.

Indulge in fresh produce. Fresh out-of-season fruits and vegetables provide a welcome taste of spring or summer in the middle of winter. Or, when your favorite fruit reaches its summertime peak, freeze it for a special holiday treat.

Lose the leftovers. Each Thanksgiving, Dr. Stern buys new plastic containers, which she promptly fills with leftovers and sends home with her guests.

Establish New Traditions

While treats such as eggnog and pecan pie will always have a place on the holiday table, keeping your new healthy perspective on eating will be tough if Thanksgiving revolves entirely around the turkey.

Starting new traditions that can help get you off the couch and away from the remote control will help. "Your metabolic rate actually drops below its baseline when you watch TV," Connolly-Schoonen says. "Anything you do is better than turning on the television."

In the spirit of activity, here are some tips for a healthier, happier holiday.

Get active. After the bird's in the oven, take a family walk or start up a game of touch football.

Be creative. Read a story aloud, sing songs, or do crafts as a family.

Volunteer. Many churches and community organizations prepare holiday meals for the homebound or the homeless. Instead of counting calories, you'll be counting your blessings.

Breakfast at Tiffany's: Eating Out

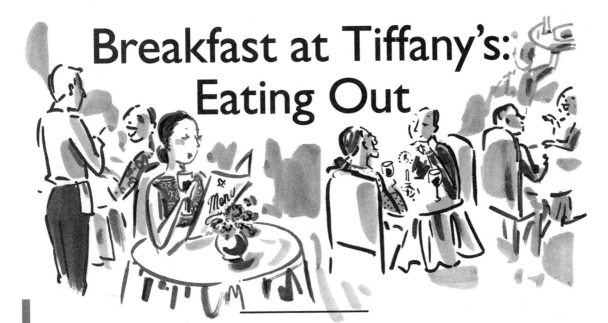

Just as Pavlov's dog was conditioned to salivate at the sound of a bell, we're conditioned to overeat at the sight of a restaurant meal.

That was fine when restaurant meals were reserved for special occasions like birthdays and anniversaries. But today, we eat out an average of four times a week. Splurge on every restaurant meal, and you're almost guaranteed to weigh more than women who rarely dine out.

"We need to get out of the mindset that every time we eat at a restaurant, it's a special occasion," says Joyce Nelsen, R.D., professor of nutrition and food safety at the Culinary Institute of America in Hyde Park, New York. "Instead, we need to think in terms of what we would eat if we were at home, then put *that* on our plates."

That's particularly important since restaurant fare can be a nutritional minefield—typically higher in fat and cholesterol and lower in calcium and fiber than homemade meals.

One of the biggest restaurant pitfalls is immense portion size. The 16-ounce steak. The ½ pound of pasta smothered with cream sauce. An 8-ounce burger. They're often two to three times larger than dietitians recommend. And we feel like we have to finish every last morsel in order to get our money's worth. "This all-you-can-eat concept is really hurting the American population," says Suzanne Vieira, R.D., director of culinary nutrition at Johnson & Wales University in Providence, Rhode Island. It has contributed to the epidemic of obesity in this country, which, in turn, is reflected in increasing rates of diabetes and heart disease, she says. Europeans, for instance, eat much smaller portions, spread their meals out over more courses, and never use doggie bags. And it shows. European women are generally thinner than we are.

Dining Out on a (Calorie) Budget

That doesn't mean you can never eat out, or that when you do, you're stuck ordering iceberg lettuce. "You shouldn't walk away from any meal feeling deprived," Nelsen says, "because that's going to sabotage your weight loss." So have a

WOMAN TO WOMAN

She Knows That Eating Out Doesn't Mean Pigging Out

Jenna Jayroe of Shreveport, Louisiana, changed the way she ate, began exercising, and lost 100 pounds. Then she landed a new job that required heavy travel, and she began eating at restaurants several times a month. Knowing that the fried foods on the menu would tempt her, she figured out how to use her new weight loss skills at restaurants, and she hasn't gained a pound in 2 years. Here is her story.

Most people choose a salad for their low-fat meal, but I hate salads unless they're drenched in blue cheese dressing, which defeats the purpose. So I skip salad entrées and eat minestrone and vegetable soups and turkey sandwiches. I always ask for mayonnaise and mustard on the side. Even though mustard is usually low-calorie, I never know if I'm going to get real mustard or some calorie-packed mustard "sauce." When I order pasta, I even ask for the red sauce on the side.

But that doesn't mean I'm not tempted by high-fat options. Once in a while, I'll be in an exciting city and want to order something that I can't get at home, so I do. I just stop eating when I'm full. One time in Las Vegas, I went to this wonderful Italian restaurant and had chicken ravioli with a rich cream sauce—*not* on the side.

I know that I can't eat high-fat dishes at every meal, but there's nothing wrong with enjoying small portions of fettuccine Alfredo or steak once in a while when you order the sauce on the side and you know how to stop eating when you're full.

I'm lucky because most of the people I dine with order healthy meals, but whenever I'm tempted to eat high-fat, I stay on track by constantly remembering my goal: to maintain my weight loss.

vents what I call unconscious eating, which is when you consume food so fast that your brain doesn't have time to let you know that you're full."

Here's how to head off huge portions.

Start with soup and a salad. Studies show that foods high in water, such as soup, are more filling, and the fiber in the salad (make it dark leafy greens for more nutritional power) will also make you feel fuller. But order a clear soup—no heavy cream—and ask for dressings on the side.

Split the entrée. Share your main course either with someone at your table or with yourself the next night. Just have the waiter wrap half before it even gets to the table.

Stick to beginnings. Order an appetizer as your main course. "Most of the time, the appetizer portions are exactly the amount of food you should be eating as an entrée," Nelsen says.

Avoid the potholes. Look out for hidden fat and calories. Go for main courses flavored with salsa, relish and chutney, or sauces derived from natural juices or vegetable reductions. "These flavorings don't have a lot of added fat, butter, or cream," says Susan Spicer, a chef at Bayona restaurant in New Orleans. Vegetarian and seafood choices are generally lower in fat, as long as they're not fried. So skip anything that has been dredged in flour or that has breading or batter. "The breading on something like eggplant Parmesan soaks up fat like a sponge," Nelsen says.

glass of wine. Split dessert with your date. And most important, take time to enjoy the food and your dining-out experience.

"One of the courses of the meal should be conversation," Vieira says. "Taking it slow pre-

Home-Style American

With all the ethnic food choices available to us today, "plain American cuisine" still ranks as our favorite. But it's chow loaded with fat and calories and focused on meat rather than healthier whole grains and vegetables. To cut through the fat trap, look for items that are grilled, marinated, or barbecued, says Nelsen.

Best Bets

- Manhattan clam chowder
- Vegetable soup
- Shrimp cocktail
- Hamburger (4 to 6 ounces uncooked weight) with lettuce, tomato, onion, barbecue sauce, and mustard (hold the cheese and mayo)
- Blackened or Cajun chicken with steamed vegetables and baked potato (hold the sour cream)
- Charbroiled pork chops
- Shrimp scampi with rice pilaf

Eating Italian

Italian restaurants are known for their breads, salads, and pastas—all healthy foods in their original states. But smother the bread with butter or olive oil, drown the salad in creamy dressings, or drench a heaping 8-ounce portion of pasta in a creamy Alfredo sauce, and give healthy a kiss good-bye.

"Pasta may be low in fat, but it still has calories," Nelsen says.

Stick with angel hair, spaghetti, linguine, fettuccine, fusille, or ziti. Pass up Alfredo, carbonara, and cream sauces in favor of marinara, mushroom, wine, and clam sauces.

Best Bets

- Minestrone
- Shrimp primavera (shrimp and vegetables in a flavored sauce)

WOMEN ASK WHY

Why do I eat more when I eat out?

Women who eat out at least six times a week take in 300 more calories and 19 more grams of fat a day than women who eat out less often. Plate size is the main culprit. Restaurants' smallest cost is food, so owners beef up entrées to make us think that we're getting a better value. A plate of pancakes at a restaurant has more than twice the recommended serving—that's 370 extra calories before the butter or syrup.

Once all that food is in front of us, it's very hard to eat only a quarter or half of it because of our "I've got to get all I've paid for" mentality. Eating out is the only time when we don't have nutrition labels, so we don't realize how much damage we're doing to our diets. Most of us can't even imagine that a focaccia club sandwich may have as much as 1,222 calories and 65 grams of fat.

You can avoid overdoing it at restaurants by requesting a nutrition guide from the manager ahead of time. If it's a chain restaurant, you can often check its Web site for nutrition tables, or write or call the corporation's customer service department. Also, listen closely to your hunger signals. It takes 20 minutes to feel full, so the slower you eat, the less you'll eat. Finally, concentrate more on your dining companion than your food.

Expert consulted
Beth Bussey, R.D.
Nutritionist
EatRight Program
University of Alabama at Birmingham

GUILT-FREE PLEASURE
Great Wines

One way to make even a plain chicken breast and steamed carrots take on an extra panache is to sip a glass of wine with it. A 3½ ounce goblet of wine has just 72 calories compared with the 201 in the can of soda that we're more likely to drink. Not only will wine improve your meal, it might even improve your health.

Studies show that red wine boosts your "good" cholesterol levels and lowers your "bad" cholesterol, thus reducing your risk of heart disease. That's because wine is chock-full of antioxidants, compounds that gobble up cell-damaging free radicals that make our cholesterol stickier than salt-water taffy.

Here's how to maximize the heart-healthy and meal-enhancing effects of wine.

Remember the region. If you like red wine, choose ones higher in antioxidants by drinking wine from the Burgundy or Bordeaux regions in France, the state of Oregon, or the Ontario region in Canada. The cool, damp climates of these areas enable grapes to stay on the vine longer, resulting in increased levels of antioxidants like resveratrol in the grape skins. If you're unsure where the grapes for your wine come from, ask a sales clerk.

Match your meal. Choose light wines for light food and full-bodied wines for rich food. For instance, pair Beaujolais with grilled vegetables, Riesling with fresh fruit, and white zinfandel with delicate fish like sole, cod, and flounder. Match Chianti with beef stir-fry, Merlot with fatty fish like salmon and tuna, and an oaky Chardonnay with vegetable stews.

Keep your money. Good wine doesn't have to be expensive. Expect to spend $7 to $15 a bottle.

Maintain moderation. One to three glasses a week is all you need to get the heart-healthy benefits of red wine. Six or more a week, studies suggest, may increase your risk for breast cancer.

- Mussels marinara
- Chicken cacciatore (make sure the chicken isn't breaded)

Chinese Choices

Whether it's takeout or dining out, Chinese menus are brimming with healthy choices—if you know where to look. Steer clear of crunchy noodles and anything sweet-and-sour (just another phrase for battered-and-fried). Choose steamed rice or vegetable fried rice over pork fried rice. And before you pick up your chopsticks, check out the menu for lower-fat choices, says Nelsen.

Best Bets
- Egg drop, hot-and-sour, wonton or Chinese vegetable soups
- Stir-fry chicken and broccoli
- Shrimp or vegetable lo mein (shrimp or vegetables over soft noodles)
- Chicken chow mein
- Vegetarian delight (steamed vegetables with tofu)
- Steamed vegetable dumplings
- One small egg roll with steamed white rice

Munching on Mexican

The basic ingredients of Mexican food—corn, chile peppers, and beans—are nourishing and low in fat and calories, as long as you're not turning them into a deep-fried-loaded-with-cheese chimichanga or chili con queso, says Nelsen. Skip the nacho chips, go for soft flour or corn tortillas over fried ones, and request black beans instead of lard-loaded refried beans. As for salsa—a tasty compilation of tomatoes, peppers, and onions—eat as much as you want. And don't worry; there are lots of great choices for an entrée.

Best Bets

- Black bean or gazpacho soups
- Chicken, shrimp, or beef fajitas (grilled and sliced chicken, shrimp, or beef wrapped in tortillas and accompanied with veggie garnishes), but skip the sour cream and Cheddar cheese garnishes
- Soft taco filled with beans, lettuce, tomatoes, and salsa topped with a sprinkle of cheese
- Chicken enchilada, hold the cheese (chicken in a softened—not fried—corn tortilla)
- Arroz con pollo (rice with chicken)
- Bean burrito with a sprinkling of cheese
- Seviche (fish marinated in lime juice)

WOMEN ASK WHY

Why are the French so thin, with all their cream sauces and rich foods?

While the French diet is high in fat and calories—think buttery croissants and rich cheeses—their lifestyle keeps them ahead of us in terms of health. Here are their secrets.

Eat at mealtime. No in-between snacking on empty calories.

Choose smaller portions. Even a four-course dinner in France provides only a quarter of the amount of food served in many American restaurants. As for those cream sauces, a French woman would eat about a tablespoon on her chicken; we'd have about a half-cup.

Limit food. No endless bread basket, all-you-can-eat salad bars or soup bowls, or 60-item buffets in France.

End with fruit. Fruit desserts, like pear tarts or poached apples, often replace rich pastries.

Eat slowly. The French are formal about food; dinner is often a 2- to 3-hour affair. Not a sandwich gulped in the car or while watching television.

Drink water. The French are more likely to drink water instead of calorie-packed juice and soda.

Walk. Most French people take public transportation and walk to and from work, shopping, and entertainment.

Expert consulted
Chris Rosenbloom, R.D., L.D., Ph.D.
Associate professor of nutrition
Georgia State University
Atlanta

Food from the Land of the Rising Sun

Japanese food is heavy on vegetables, rice, seaweed, and seafood and light on meat, making it one of the healthiest ethnic cuisines around, says Vieira. Just stay away from tempura, katsu, and agemono. Translation: fried.

Best Bets

- Miso (soy bean soup) or Sui Mono (clear soup)
- Sushi (rice rolls filled with raw fish or vegetables and wrapped in seaweed paper)

BATTLE OF THE BULGING RESTAURANT PLATES

"Do you make a pasta bowl that holds 80 ounces?" Restaurant-supply companies aren't looking for a family-style serving bowl when they ask that question of the Homer Laughlin China Company in Newell, West Virginia. They're after a single-serving plate, reflecting the trend towards gargantuan servings.

Plates are not only bigger but also deeper, says J. Parry, Laughlin's design director. "Some of the plates are like soup bowls now," he says. And the standard dinner plate? It's now a salad plate at some restaurants.

The reason is that with American consumers spending about half their food dollars dining out, we want value—that is, quantity—for our money. Even beverage glasses are increasing from about 14 ounces to as many as 24 ounces.

So will plates just keep mushrooming until something (or someone) explodes? Not likely.

For that to happen, restaurant tables would have to get bigger, says Parry. And that would mean fewer tables in the restaurant, which translates to fewer customers—and less income.

- Sashimi (sliced raw fish served with radish, horseradish, ginger, or soy sauce)
- Yakitori Don (broiled chicken with rice)
- Shakenabe (salmon and vegetables in soy bean broth)
- Sunomono (seafood or raw vegetables tossed with a sweet-and-sour vinaigrette)

Tasty Thai

Thai cuisine relies on exotic ingredients like lemongrass and curry to create unique dishes that manage at the same time to be both spicy and sweet. Dishes often feature fruits like mango, papaya, and pineapple, while vegetables, jasmine

rice, and seafood also take center stage. Skip anything made with coconut oil or coconut butter, which is high in saturated fat, says Vieira.

Best Bets
- Tom yum koong (clear-broth lemongrass soup with shrimp)
- Crystal noodle (chicken noodle with vegetables)
- Green curry with chicken
- Thai chicken (chicken sautéed with cashews, onions, mushrooms, pineapple, scallions, and chili)
- Garlic shrimp
- Beef basil (sautéed beef flavored with hot basil leaves, fresh hot pepper, mushrooms, and red pepper)
- Vegetable boat (string beans, asparagus, zucchini, onions, and mushrooms in Thai spices)

French Feasting

French food fairly bursts with fat. Cream sauces. Duck legs roasted in their own drippings. Pâté de foie gras. To get around all this fattening fare, look for entrées that are lightly sautéed and avoid anything with aïoli (a garlic mayonnaise made of eggs and oil), béarnaise sauce (cream sauce made with eggs and butter), or beurre blanc (white sauce that's heavy on the butter), says Vieira.

Best Bets
- Bouillabaisse (seafood stew)
- Ratatouille (side dish of vegetables simmered in olive oil, garlic, and herbs)
- Crudités (marinated vegetables such as celery root, red cabbage, cucumber, leeks, and tomatoes served raw or lightly cooked)

- Rouille (spicy sauce served with fish)
- En papillote (usually fish baked or steamed in parchment paper)
- Coulis (fruit or vegetable puree served over poultry or meat)

Indian Fare

Indian cuisine is big on vegetables, basmati rice, and sauces based on legumes like chickpeas. Just stay away from korma (cream sauce) and dishes made with coconut. "Coconut oil is the most saturated oil known to man," Nelsen says. Also pass on the pappadam—fried lentil chips— and go with chapati or nan breads instead of the fried poori or paratha.

Best Bets

- Mulligatawny (lentil, vegetable, and spice soup)
- Dahl rasam (pepper soup with lentils)
- Dahl (a spicy lentil sauce)
- Raita (side dish mixture of yogurt, cucumber, and onion)
- Vegetable biryani or pullao (similar to rice pilaf)
- Tandoori chicken or fish (marinated in spices and slow-roasted in a clay oven)
- Chicken or shrimp saag (spinach)

- Saag panir (a spinach dish featuring cheese made with milk and lemon juice)
- Chicken or fish masala (a red sauce generally lower in fat)

Save Room for Dessert

Indulging in dessert won't blow your diet, as long as you make smart choices. If you must have that chocolate torte, split it with someone at your table or have it only on very special occasions, suggests Susan Lifrieri-Lowry, chef coordinator and pastry chef at the French Culinary Institute in New York City. Even better, satisfy your sweet tooth with one of these delectable, relatively low-fat and low-calorie desserts.

Best Bets

- Vacherin (a meringue shell filled with fruit or sorbet)
- Fruit tart
- Fruit crisp
- Baked apple
- Poached pear
- Fruit soufflé
- Roasted fruit or compote in a phyllo shell
- Crème caramel or flan (rather than crème brûlée)
- Sorbet

The Times, They Are A-Changing: New Research in Medicine

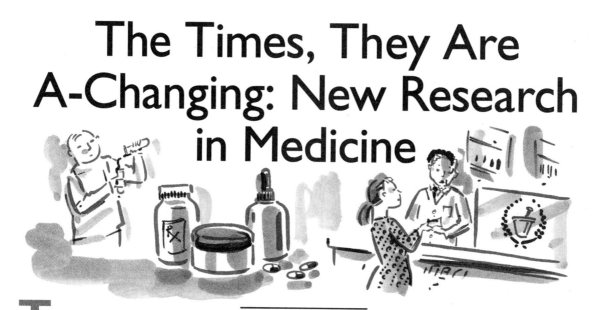

To any woman who has wrestled with the scale, a prescription for a weight loss drug that can quickly melt pounds away sounds like a miracle. Oh, the possibilities! No more "dieter's platters" of cottage cheese and peach halves. No more sweaty 5:00 P.M. aerobics classes. And all the chocolate ice cream we can eat. Sounds too good to be true!

Which, of course, immediately tells you that it is.

"The reality is that anyone who takes medication to lose weight will end up doing the same things that anyone else does to lose weight: namely, altering their eating habits and exercising once the medications are discontinued. That's the part most people don't realize," says Evelyn L. Lewis, M.D., director of the university health center at the Uniformed Services University of the Health Sciences in Bethesda, Maryland, and a weight loss researcher. "When the medications are discontinued, the majority of patients tend to regain the weight they've lost—and more—because they haven't changed their lifestyle behaviors."

As helpful as weight loss medications can be, they're not the proverbial magic bullet that we all wish they were. They're really tools that help control appetite and help keep us motivated as we pursue our weight loss goals.

New Thinking, New Treatments

In the past, physicians have been reluctant to prescribe drugs for weight loss. "People used to think that losing weight was a matter of willpower," explains Caroline M. Apovian, M.D., director of the Nutrition and Weight Management Center at Boston Medical Center and associate professor of medicine at Boston University School of Medicine. "Many doctors felt the same way."

But physicians and researchers are beginning to revise their thinking.

Discoveries of hormones and proteins that influence everything from our appetites to our metabolism have opened new worlds in obesity research and potential treatments. At the same time, despite a never-ending parade of diets, Americans are in the middle of what researchers and doctors call an obesity epidemic.

Dr. Apovian believes that it is vital to the control of this epidemic that medical professionals treat obesity as a chronic disease like diabetes or high blood pressure instead of writing it off as a symptom of weak willpower.

"What's so different about taking drugs for obesity?" Dr. Apovian asks. "People with hypertension take drugs. People with diabetes take drugs. Why is it that obese people can't take drugs to manage their disease, like orlistat (Xenical), which keeps your body from absorbing fat from your meals, lowers blood pressure, lowers cholesterol, and helps you lose weight. That's three bangs for your buck."

Although the first generation of weight loss drugs comprised mostly amphetamines, which can be highly habit-forming, the current generation tends to be much safer. "When the amphetamines came out, no one really understood their truly addictive nature," says Denise Bruner, M.D., president of the American Society of Bariatric Physicians and a physician practicing in Arlington, Virginia. Now, if your doctor prescribes medication to help you lose weight, she'll probably give you one of three options: orlistat, a fat-blocker; Sibutramine (Meridia), which helps you feel full faster; or

WOMEN ASK WHY
Can some medicines really make me fat?

Yes. Some medications, such as those that treat mental illness, work through a mechanism in your central nervous system that affects the concentrations of chemicals in the brain. As a result, they can affect your appetite or your feelings of satiety, the "fullness" that tells you when to stop eating. If you're taking one of the older tricyclic antidepressants, for example, you may notice an increased appetite. The same thing happens with lithium, typically prescribed for depression or mania, or antipsychotic drugs such as clozapine, often prescribed for schizophrenia.

Other drugs actually affect how fat is stored or distributed in your body. Corticosteroids (typically prescribed for conditions such as rheumatoid arthritis, allergies, or asthma) not only increase your appetite but also shift where your body stores fat. Instead of depositing it in your arms or legs, your body moves it to your torso. Even worse, this centrally stored fat puts you at greater risk for cardiovascular disease, and these medications put you at greater risk for diabetes.

If you have diabetes, you typically gain weight when you get your blood sugar under control with medications. With uncontrolled diabetes, calories are not being stored; they're going out in the urine. Once your insulin levels are stabilized, you return your body's energy balance to what it would have been if diabetes hadn't intervened. Wait until you get your diabetes under control before you address your weight.

Finally, if you're considering a hormonal contraceptive such as Depo-Provera, be prepared to feel hungry; the progestin in this drug probably stimulates appetite. Many women gain 5 to 10 pounds in their first year on this birth control.

If you think that your prescription is making you gain weight, talk to your doctor about alternatives.

Expert consulted
Julie Oki, Pharm.D.
Associate professor of medicine
University of Missouri–Kansas City School of
Medicine

Phentermine (Phentride), an appetite suppressant.

Should You or Shouldn't You?

If you've tried diet after diet with limited success, you may be thinking, "I'm the perfect candidate for a diet pill!" But the decision to take weight loss drugs depends on multiple factors. Your dieting history is important, of course; but so is your weight, your health, and most important, your willingness to change your lifestyle.

"These drugs are not so potent that the patient doesn't have to do her part," cautions Mary Wangsness, M.D., a bariatric physician in St. Paul, Minnesota.

In addition, they're drugs, which means that they carry risks as well as benefits. Before you take a single pill, your doctor will want to give you a thorough medical screening, checking for everything from heart problems to high cholesterol. She'll also calculate your body mass index (BMI) and ask about your health. Doctors generally reserve weight loss drugs for those of us who are severely overweight, with a BMI of 30 if we're otherwise healthy, or 27, if we have conditions such as diabetes or high blood pressure, which can be helped by losing weight. So, if you're just trying to lose those last 10 pounds before your 25-year high school reunion, forget anti-obesity meds; it's back to the treadmill for you.

Even if you meet the BMI requirements, you

WHAT'S WRONG WITH FEN-PHEN ANYWAY?

To many dieters, the drug combo fen-phen seemed like the answer to a lifelong prayer. Thanks to the appetite suppressant phentermine (the "phen" of the famous pharmaceutical combination), they simply didn't feel hungry. When they did eat, fenfluramine (a.k.a. "fen"), with its serotonin-boosting effects, helped them feel full sooner.

"My patients on fen-phen didn't care about food. Many had to force themselves to eat," remembers Mary Wangsness, M.D., a bariatric physician in St. Paul, Minnesota. "For many people who had struggled with their weight, fen-phen seemed to be a miracle drug."

But fen-phen, which was never approved for combination therapy by the FDA, was a short-lived miracle with serious consequences.

In 1997, researchers found that some fen-phen users had leaky heart valves, a condition called valvular heart disease. As a result, drug manufacturers pulled fenfluramine and a related drug, dexfenfluramine, from the market. The suspicion was that fenfluramine's effect on serotonin was to blame. Phentermine, which is considered safe when used alone, remains in use.

To compensate for the blood that leaks back into your heart through the damaged valve, explains Christina Wee,

mustn't think that you can start using that treadmill as a plant holder or that you can fill your freezer with full-fat ice cream. Your doctor may be writing the prescription, but she'll expect you to be an active participant in your weight loss efforts. "Patients sometimes think that between me and the Meridia, the job will get done. Well, it just doesn't work that way," Dr. Wangsness says. The drugs may give you a jump start on your weight loss, but you need to adopt a healthier lifestyle that will work in concert with your medication.

M.D., instructor of medicine at Harvard Medical School, your heart must work harder to ensure that enough blood reaches the rest of your body. "Over time, that adds up to a lot of stress on the heart, and the heart can grow weaker," she says.

Other fen-phen users developed pulmonary hypertension, or high blood pressure in the blood vessels of the lungs, which makes it hard for the heart and lungs to provide the oxygenated blood we need to live.

There is some good news if you took fen-phen: Preliminary evidence from studies suggests that heart valves damaged by the drug combo may heal themselves, says Dr. Wee, although she emphasizes that the jury is still out on this matter.

Even if you haven't experienced any symptoms, that doesn't mean you're home-free. "With fen-phen, by the time you realize you have valvular heart disease, it may already be severe," says Dr. Wee. If you used fen-phen, talk to your doctor. She may want to screen you for valve problems, especially if you used the drug for longer than 6 months or expect to have dental work or surgery in the near future. As a precaution, you may want to ask about preventive antibiotics before any invasive procedures. Otherwise, bacteria that enter your bloodstream may become lodged in a damaged valve that you didn't know you had.

Orlistat: Stop Fat Before It Starts

"A moment on the lips, a lifetime on the hips," the old saying goes. Unless, that is, you're taking orlistat, one of the newest kids on the weight loss block.

What it does: A weight loss drug known as a lipase inhibitor, orlistat prevents your body from absorbing the fat in the foods you eat by as much as 30 percent. In one study, men and women on the drug lost an average of nearly 20 pounds in the first year of treatment. Just imagine: You could eat cheesecake, French fries, potato chips, and more, yet only ingest two-thirds of those fat calories. It sounds like the ultimate wonder drug for our fast-food society . . . until the "gastrointestinal events" begin.

What to expect: "If you go to McDonald's and order a Big Mac while you're taking orlistat, you're in for a big shock," Dr. Wangsness says. It's great that your body is absorbing only 70 percent of those fat calories, but that other 30 percent has to go somewhere. Which leads to the most common side effects: oily or fatty stools, oily spotting, and increased urgency in bowel movements.

Make it work for you: If you're eating responsibly and sticking to a diet with 30 percent fat or less (which is what most nutritionists recommend anyway), you don't need to worry about "orlistat's revenge." "It's really a behavior modification drug," explains Dr. Wangsness. "Most people are afraid of the side effects, so they watch their diets." As a result, you develop better eating habits, lose weight, and often improve your cholesterol levels and blood pressure.

One more thing: When orlistat eliminates that 30 percent of the fat, you're also losing valuable fat-soluble vitamins such as A, D, E, and K. It's recommended that you take a multivitamin whenever you are on a weight loss program.

Sibutramine: Feel Full Faster

Perhaps potato chips and other high-fat foods hold no charm for you. They don't fill you up.

Then again, neither does anything else. No matter how much you eat, you never seem to feel full.

You might want to talk to your doctor about sibutramine (Meridia).

What it does: Sibutramine prevents the intake of serotonin and norepinephrine—mood-lifting hormones—into your appetite center, thereby increasing your feeling of fullness. It also increases your heart rate and blood pressure, making this drug a poor choice for someone with heart problems or uncontrolled high blood pressure.

What to expect: You'll still feel hungry, but thanks to these increased levels of circulating serotonin and norepinephrine, you'll feel full faster and, hopefully, eat less. You won't lose dramatic amounts of weight; in one study, people lost an average of 10 to 14 pounds in a year, depending on how much sibutramine they took.

Make it work for you: Although sibutramine is considered an appetite suppressant, you'll still get hungry; you just won't need to eat as much to feel sated.

One more thing: If you're currently taking any drugs for depression, it's necessary to check with your physician before taking sibutramine.

Phentermine: Reduce Your Hunger Pangs

Phentermine grabbed headlines in 1997 as the second syllable of the popular diet drug combo fen-phen when fenfluramine—the "fen" part—was recalled.

LEPTIN: BIG PROMISES, LITTLE REALITY

When researchers discovered leptin in 1995, they thought they had solved the obesity equation. Leptin, a hormone found in fat cells, seemed to influence both appetite and metabolism, leading to weight loss in obese mice injected with the substance. Researchers hoped that leptin could do the same for people, helping them manage obesity as people with diabetes rely on insulin to control their condition. But leptin (from the Greek word for thin) had other plans.

"Leptin is probably the greatest discovery in obesity in this century, but it's probably not going to help women lose weight," says Eleftheria Maratos-Flier, M.D., associate professor of medicine at Harvard Medical School and an investigator at the Joslin Diabetes Center in Boston.

That's because its role in regulating body weight has proven more complex and subtle than researchers initially thought. Instead of controlling appetite or metabolism directly, leptin primarily tells our brains how much energy—or fat stores—our bodies have. Thanks to these leptin signals, our brains decide whether we have enough body fat to perform the "extras" of life, such as menstruation or carrying a baby. So, the amount of leptin in our blood generally corresponds to our percentage of body

Used independently, phentermine remains a safe and effective weight loss drug for short-term use.

What it does: Considered a "second generation" obesity drug, phentermine chemically resembles the amphetamines that doctors initially prescribed for weight loss. It raises your blood pressure, increases your heart rate, and suppresses your appetite.

What to expect: For women who feel deprived when they diet, ravenous as opposed to hungry, and unable to control their appetites, phentermine can help.

fat. If we're thin, we have little leptin; if we're heavy, we have lots.

But, if we're born without any leptin (a rare genetic disorder), this body-weight/leptin ratio gets out of whack. Without any leptin in our systems, the brain thinks we're starving and tries to save us. Our metabolism slows down. We eat uncontrollably. We become huge. Give us leptin, though, and the pounds drop off as we start eating and burning calories normally. No wonder obesity researchers were so excited about this hormone.

Give a normal overweight person leptin, though, and you won't see such dramatic effects. Men and women who received the highest doses of leptin in one major study lost an average of only 15½ pounds in 6 months—less than a pound a week. "Leptin hasn't worked well as a therapy because most people have pretty high leptin levels," Dr. Maratos-Flier explains. "When you give them more, it doesn't really do anything."

Leptin may eventually prove more effective in preventing weight regain in people who have dieted, Dr. Maratos-Flier suggests. Raising leptin levels in a woman's blood could trick her brain into thinking that she hasn't lost the weight, protecting her newly svelte figure (and reduced leptin levels) from being interpreted by her brain as a sign of starvation.

Make it work for you: Just as orlistat and sibutramine users need to develop healthier eating and exercise habits, so, too, do those taking phentermine. The effects of phentermine, like many weight loss drugs, seem to plateau around 6 months, so if you haven't been exercising and eating right, you will probably experience problems keeping the weight off.

One more thing: If you're a former fen-phen patient who wants to try anti-obesity medications again, you might consider phentermine. Sibutramine may not be as effective for former fen-phen users, Dr. Wangsness says, but a trial would certainly be worthwhile because in many situations, it works very well.

The Next Generation?

If you've tried all three of these medications with no success, don't throw up your hands in despair. Obesity researchers are constantly discovering more and more about the intricate relationship between the brain and weight. Soon they may be able to create a new generation of weight loss treatments that target specific mechanisms in the brain that lead to obesity.

One of those mechanisms is leptin, a hormone that tells our brains how much body fat we have, allowing the brain to regulate how much we eat and how many calories we can burn.

"Leptin was the elephant in the room of obesity, and we didn't even know it existed until recently," says Sheila Collins, Ph.D., associate professor at Duke University Medical Center in Durham, North Carolina. Now researchers just have to figure out how to successfully manipulate the complex hormone.

It may be a while before any new discovery leads to a safer and more effective obesity treatment, however. Weight gain is a very complex process, and we just don't know how all the pieces of the puzzle fit together yet. For now, the "wiring diagram is still a little fuzzy," Dr. Collins says. "Like diabetes, the problem contributing to and causing obesity is not just in one place." It involves multiple proteins, hormones, and body chemicals that influence

REAL-LIFE SCENARIO

She Went Off Her High Blood Pressure Medication because She Thinks It's Making Her Gain Weight

When Kylie first learned that she had high blood pressure, she was upset and frightened. How could a woman of 38, especially one who has remained so healthy, trim, and fit, have that kind of problem unless there was something seriously wrong? Her doctor's reassurance that she could control it with medication calmed her. But after a few months of taking pills, her blood pressure is down, but her weight is up. She'd rather deal with the high blood pressure than get fat, so now she has gone off her medicine. Has she done the right thing?

Kylie needs to talk to her doctor. Her physician needs to clearly understand her concerns and the reasons why she has stopped taking her medication.

Sometimes beta-blockers and other centrally-acting hypertensives can make you feel more sedated or sluggish, especially when you start the therapy. Because the medication blocks the adrenaline response in the heart, it's tough to get your heart rate up, even when exercising vigorously. It may be the decreased energy expenditure that's making Kylie gain weight.

If that's affecting Kylie's quality of life, she needs to talk to her physician. Beta-blockers can be truly lifesaving depending on why they're prescribed. If you've had a heart attack and you've been given a beta-blocker, it could save your life. But, if Kylie isn't tolerating this drug well, there are lots of alternative blood pressure medications available. She could ask about diuretics, which in low doses aren't likely to cause weight gain, or ACE inhibitors, which relax the blood vessels.

Regardless of what medication she chooses with her doctor, Kylie needs to take it as directed. High blood pressure is a big deal; a stroke is far more debilitating than some weight gain or sluggishness.

Expert consulted
Julie Oki, Pharm.D
Associate professor of medicine
University of Missouri–Kansas City School
    of Medicine

our appetites, percentage of body fat, satiety, metabolism, and more. Metabolism alone has so many checks and balances that it may be impossible to alter one body process intentionally without affecting another that negates the original efforts. The answer to such a complicated question might involve multiple therapies.

The bottom line? Don't postpone your weight loss plans to wait for the next miracle drug. Our bodies have evolved over centuries, surviving the physical exertions of the hunter-gatherer days to confront today's fast-food society, "where it takes a calorie to roll down your window at the McDonald's drive-thru and get 3,000 calories to eat," Dr. Apovian says.

Regardless of what weight loss drug our doctors may prescribe for us in the new millennium, Dr. Collins says, "there will always be a place for diet and exercise."

Doin' What Comes Naturally: Supplements

Intellectually, we know the kind of lifestyle changes we need to make to lose weight: Move more and eat fewer calories. But in our hearts, we lust after the easy solution. The pill we can pop. The cream we can rub. The shake we can down. After all, we think, we've perfected the art of 24-hour shopping without leaving the house; why can't we figure out a pain-free weight loss method?

Manufacturers understand our longing. That's why dozens of dietary supplements crowd store shelves, enticing us with whispered (and shouted) promises to sate our hunger, speed our metabolism, and absorb fat before it has a chance to find our thighs and butt.

While old friends like meal-replacement drinks and heart-racing drugstore pills are still out there, the hottest area in weight loss today is in so-called natural supplements containing ingredients like ephedra, chromium picolinate, hydroxycitric acid, and chitosan.

"Natural supplements are presumed to be safe because they come from nature in their original form," says Laurie Fan, director of content management at BioValidity.com and publisher of the *BioNutritional Encyclopedia* and other life science databases on the Internet.

And some *are* safe, says Gail Mahady, Ph.D., assistant professor of pharmacognosy at the University of Illinois at Chicago. "But some of the most potent toxins on the face of the Earth come from plants."

Not to mention the fact that most of them don't work as manufacturers promise they will.

Ephedra

Of all the "natural" weight loss substances, the herb ephedra is the most controversial. Commonly known by its Chinese name, *ma huang*, it has been used in China for more than 5,000 years to treat bronchial asthma and other upper respiratory conditions. But, ironically, never for weight loss.

Yet in this country, it's found in hundreds of diet supplements, powders, drinks, and diet bars along with other stimulants that claim to decrease appetite, raise metabolism, and burn fat.

Its active ingredient, ephedrine, stimulates cardiovascular and central nervous systems, which

Why don't I feel full until after I've overeaten?

Chances are, you're eating too fast, skipping breakfast or lunch, or waiting too long to eat between meals.

Wolfing down meals means there isn't enough time for a message from the chemicals in your stomach to reach the chemicals in your brain, signaling that you're full. Like a bad phone connection, this communication takes about 20 minutes to go through. Thus, you keep eating, only to realize that you're way past comfortable when that 20 minutes hits.

If you're skipping meals or waiting too long between meals, you have another problem: You're ravenous. So when you hit the table, your self-control disappears like an ice cube in August. By the time that signal saying "enough" hits your brain, you've eaten tomorrow's leftovers.

Here's how to break the cycle.

Eat regularly. If you might miss a meal, carry some healthy snacks like peanut butter and apples or low-fat yogurt with you. Make sure that your snacks include protein— it keeps you full longer than carbohydrates alone.

Eat between meals. Who says you should eat only three times a day? Try those same snacks mentioned above even if you don't miss a meal so that you're eating something every 3 to 4 hours. This keeps your blood sugar stabilized and prevents overeating at the next meal.

Slow down. Chew your food slowly. Talk to people or put your knife and fork down between bites. Get up and walk around the house twice before you reach for seconds.

Get out of the kitchen. Instead of eating where the food is, take your plate to another room. Suddenly, getting seconds might be too much of an effort.

Expert consulted
Michele Trankina, Ph.D.
Nutritional consultant
Professor of biological sciences
St. Mary's University of San Antonio

may speed heart rates, boost blood pressure, and induce nervousness, insomnia, headaches, or dizziness. In high doses, it may contribute to stroke, heart attack, seizures, and even death, says Dr. Mahady.

And its effects on weight loss are disappointing.

That's why some manufacturers combine it with caffeine and aspirin to make thermogenic supplements called E-C-A. In fact, ephedrine and caffeine do work together to increase metabolism and decrease appetite, says Carla Wolper, R.D., a nutritionist at the Obesity Research Center at St. Luke's–Roosevelt Hospital Center in New York City. She cautions, however, that adding aspirin to the mix can cause stomach problems in some people. And, because caffeine and ephedra are both stimulants, you eventually build up a tolerance to them.

In at least one 6-week study, the E-C-A combination appeared to work. Those taking the mixture three times a day with meals lost 9 pounds compared with the $1\frac{1}{2}$ pounds lost by the group taking a placebo.

One problem: Like many ephedra-based supplements, the mixture may cause irregular heartbeats, anxiety, and jitteriness. Since 1994, the FDA has received more than 800 complaints from people experiencing side effects from taking ephedra-based products.

Talk with your doctor before taking any over-the-counter weight loss aids. And since ephedra can create so many serious health problems, you should use it only under the guidance of a qualified practitioner.

Chromium Picolinate

Several studies suggest that this supplement, a form of the mineral chromium, builds muscle and reduces fat. Chromium assists in deriving energy from carbohydrates and fats, improving your body's response to the hormone insulin so that your blood sugar levels remain steady.

Weight loss studies are mixed, however. One reason for the disparate results may have to do with the way studies are designed. Some researchers think that the supplement works only if your diet is already chromium-deficient. Others say that it depends on the type of chromium used, dosage, and length of time it's taken.

Still others conclude that it just doesn't work as well as the mainstays of weight loss: exercise and a low-fat, high-fiber diet.

They do agree on one thing, however: It's safe.

Recommended dose: 400 to 600 micrograms per day. Don't expect immediate results; you'll need to take it for nearly 6 months before you see a change, says Richard A. Anderson, Ph.D., lead scientist at the USDA Human Nutrition Research Center in Beltsville, Maryland. Doses above 200 micrograms should be taken under medical supervision.

Chitosan

This fiberlike substance comes from the shells of lobster, crab, shrimp, and insects. It suppos-

WOMEN ASK WHY

If I drink 48 ounces of water a day, why don't I gain 48 ounces when I jump on the scale?

With 60 percent of our bodies made up of water, it's no surprise that nearly every cell needs the wet stuff to survive. So as quick as you take in fluid, your body uses it up, discarding what it doesn't need in the form of urine and perspiration. The amount discarded varies due to factors such as physical exertion, climate, and your weight.

When you first go on a high-protein, low-carbohydrate diet, you may notice an initial weight reduction, but it's mainly water. When protein is broken down, more water is created, which your kidneys then have to filter and get rid of. Your kidneys also have to work overtime to get rid of excess protein, which is why these diets may cause kidney damage.

Expert consulted
Michele Trankina, Ph.D.
Nutritional consultant
Professor of biological sciences
St. Mary's University of San Antonio

edly helps you lose weight by absorbing fat in your digestive tract for, ahem, elimination before it can glom onto your hips and thighs.

Sounds good in theory. But here's the problem: Chitosan not only binds fat but also essential vitamins that need fat to get into your cells. We're talking about vitamins like A, D, E, and K as well as important phytonutrients like carotenoids that protect against cancer and other chronic diseases, says Michele Trankina, Ph.D., nutritional consultant and professor of biological sciences at St. Mary's University of San Antonio.

Send all that on a one-way trip out of your body, and you may end up short on vital nutrients.

"People may be tempted to take more of these vitamins to make up for what they lose through the chitosan," Dr. Trankina says. Don't. "Some fat-soluble vitamins can be toxic—and even fatal—taken in high doses."

And it's not even certain that chitosan really helps with weight loss. Of three European studies examining chitosan's effects, only one found any benefit. In that very small study, 10 overweight men and women lost an average of 9 pounds after taking 2,000 milligrams of chitosan and eating a 1,200 calorie-a-day diet for 4 weeks. Another 10 people who received a placebo lost 6 pounds.

It's possible that the biggest contributor was the very low calorie diet, for when researchers tried a similar study without restricting calories, no one lost any weight.

Pyruvate

Pyruvate is a natural substance resulting from the breakdown of carbohydrates in our bodies. It's found in the blood, heart, brain, and liver. It's even found in food, such as red apples, red wine, Cheddar and provolone cheese, bananas, and garlic.

To date, research shows that pyruvate is a safe and effective weight loss supplement when combined with a healthy diet and regular exercise. It's a natural metabolism booster, and it prevents your body from producing fat, says Judith E. Arch, R.D., a bionutritionist at the University of Pittsburgh General Clinical Research Center.

In one study, overweight women who took pyruvate lost 37 percent more weight and 48 percent more body fat than those taking a placebo. The supplement seems to help even without a low-calorie diet, says Ronald Stanko, M.D., associate professor at the University of

Pittsburgh Medical Center and principle author of pyruvate studies.

Another pyruvate benefit is that it preserves muscle mass—your own fat-burning system—which many women lose when they rely on low-calorie, no-exercise programs for weight loss, Dr. Stanko says.

Sounds almost too good to be true—and it may be.

"You can't just rely on the pill," Arch says. "You really have to eat a healthy diet rich in fruits, vegetables, and whole grains. And you should keep you activity level up. Otherwise, your expectations will be a lot higher than your results, and you'll be disappointed."

Recommended dose: 4 to 6 grams a day, according to Dr. Stanko.

Guaraná

Nicknamed "zoom" because of its tendency to perk you up faster than a triple espresso, guaraná is a dried paste made from the crushed seeds of *Paullinia cupana*, a woody shrub native to Brazil and Uruguay.

It gets its name from the Guaranis South American Indians, who have used it for thousands of years as an aphrodisiac, diarrhea treatment, and for sustenance during long fasts.

Today, you're most likely to find it in South American carbonated drinks, where its high caffeine content provides a quick jolt. In this country, however, we've grabbed onto it for weight loss.

In truth, we might be better off with that espresso. It has more caffeine for the money, and it doesn't contain high concentrations of tannin, which may pose a long-term cancer risk.

Plus, there really aren't any published studies showing that guaraná works for weight loss.

Its use is associated with possible side effects like anxiety, nervousness, insomnia, stomach upset, headaches, and heart palpitations. It's often sold in combination with ephedra and other stimulants, which usually make these symptoms worse and may cause other health problems. Because it contains twice the caffeine found in coffee, long-term use of excessive amounts isn't recommended because it stimulates the nervous system. It can also irritate the gastrointestinal tract. Avoid guaraná if you have heart disease or if you're sensitive to caffeine or are pregnant or nursing.

Hydroxycitric Acid

Called HCA for short, most hydroxycitric acid comes from the tropical fruit *Garcinia cambogia*, commonly known as the brindall berry. It's a modified form of citric acid, which turns the food we eat into the calories we burn or store as fat.

Basically, HCA prevents your body from making fat by blocking a certain enzyme that normally converts citric acid to fat. Animal studies support these claims, but they haven't lived up to their promise in humans.

For example, when researchers at St. Luke's–Roosevelt Hospital gave a group of overweight men and women 1,500 milligrams of HCA a day for 12 weeks, they each lost an average of 9 pounds. A placebo group lost 7—not a significant difference. Both were on high-fiber, low-calorie diets anyway.

WOMAN TO WOMAN

Good-bye Weight Loss Supplements, Hello Exercise

Although her son was already 16, Donna Wetterau of Coplay, Pennsylvania, was still trying to lose her postbaby weight gain of 60 pounds. Throughout the years, Donna, 50, had followed a vicious cycle of yo-yo dieting, experimenting with numerous over-the-counter and prescription weight loss supplements. By age 47, Donna was 100 pounds overweight and understandably depressed. Then she discovered the wonders of regular exercise and healthy eating. Here's her story.

I began using weight loss supplements to curb my appetite when I was 25 and continued until I was 45. I tried meal-replacement drinks and powdered fruit-juice mixes. Over-the-counter supplements didn't work. Prescription pills helped me shed some pounds, but only during the 6 months I was allowed to take them. After that, my doctor said that my body would build up a tolerance, and I could become addicted to the pills.

By the time I was 47, I was facing high blood pressure and diabetes. So I decided to take one more stab at losing weight—the right way.

I began walking 30 minutes a day. Later, I joined a gym and found a personal trainer who showed me how to combine daily treadmill walking and cycling with weight training. I walked 3 miles a day, 6 days a week and weight trained 3 days a week.

Once I started working out, I began to eat healthy, low-fat foods, reduced-calorie snacks, and smaller portion sizes. I stopped skipping meals and started eating breakfast, lunch, and dinner. And I limited high-fat foods and snacks to once or twice a month.

So far, I've lost 80 pounds and gone down eight dress sizes in less than 2 years, and I hope to lose another 20 pounds. I never thought I'd lose all of this weight, especially at my age. But now that I've done it, I know that I'll be sticking with exercise and healthy eating for the rest of my life. Finally, I'm in control of my body.

WHO REGULATES THE DIET-SUPPLEMENT INDUSTRY?

No one, really. In 1994, Congress passed the Dietary Supplement Health and Education Act (DSHEA), putting supplements like ephedra and pyruvate in the same category as food. Thus, although they fall under the jurisdiction of the FDA, manufacturers can market their products without prior approval from the FDA, without any premarketing testing, and without even proving that the product is safe. There's also no manufacturing oversight, as there is with prescription drugs, to ensure quality. So no one is actually checking that the active ingredient from the herb was used in the preparation or that the dosage described on the bottle is actually in the pill.

Right now, people are on their own. And some of the worst offenders are in the weight loss industry because there's such demand. People still want the magic bullet.

Expert consulted
Ruth Kava, R.D., Ph.D.
Director of nutrition
American Council on Science and Health
New York City

"There's really no evidence proving that HCA actually works," Dr. Mahady says. "So at this point, I wouldn't recommend buying it.

Meal-Replacement Drinks

Ah, if only we didn't have to prepare, cook, and clean up meals. By now, we'd be fluent in three languages and have written that bestseller. Enter meal-replacement drinks like Ultra Slim Fast and Nestle Sweet Success.

The good news: They're enormous time-savers, they don't contain any harmful drugs or herbs, and they come in a variety of flavors, including the pièce de résistance: chocolate.

The bad news: They might not make you feel any less hungry.

Full of vitamins and minerals yet low in fat, their marketing claims tout them as weight loss–inducing substitutes for breakfast and lunch. And it's true; if you occasionally substitute a 200-calorie drink for a 1,000-calorie pastrami sandwich, you will lose weight eventually. But Wolper is concerned that using diet drinks regularly causes you to miss the benefits of eating a wide range of food.

"I don't recommend any woman staying on this plan for any length of time," Wolper says. "You'll miss out on a wide variety of foods that contain important nutrients."

Diet Pills

Appetite suppressants such as Dexatrim and Acutrim have been available over the counter for decades. Their main ingredient, phenylpropanolamine, related to amphetamine, is known to suppress appetite.

"It works by stimulating certain chemicals in your brain that tell your appetite center to take a nap," Wolper says.

Thus, it will reduce your appetite—for a while. Eventually, however, you'll build up a tolerance to the drug, and its effects will wear off.

Supplement warning: Phenylpropanolamine can cause nervousness, dizziness, insomnia, heart palpitations, and headache. It has also been associated with stroke, seizures, heart attacks, arrhythmia, psychosis, and even death.

Steer clear if you're being treated for depression, an eating disorder, if you're pregnant or nursing, have high blood pressure, diabetes, thyroid problems, or heart disease.

PART FOUR

The Beat
Goes On

The Long and Winding Road: The Cycles in a Woman's Life

When many of us hit our forties, all the birthday presents and cards in the world can't disguise one significant fact: We've gained weight. No longer can we get away with eating that extra slice of pepperoni pizza on Monday, that double cheeseburger and large fries on Friday, or that chocolate ice cream sundae on Saturday.

In our twenties, however, ahhhh, that's when we could eat. Late-night parties where the four food groups were nachos, potato chips, sour cream dip, and beer. Decadent Sunday brunches of chocolate chip pancakes with a side of bacon. Then we'd slip into another size 4 pair of jeans and head out for a day of antiquing or roller blading or any of the other thousand things we used to do before we had kids and soccer games and husbands and houses and dogs to fill our weekends. If we gained a few pounds, no problem. A couple of nights at the gym, a jog along the beach, and poof! The extra weight was gone.

No more. Now, in addition to the fullness of our lives, we've added the fullness of our figures,

mainly around our hips, butts, thighs, and pouchy stomachs.

Even more discouraging: Those pounds seem stuck to us with Superglue.

And so we moan the eternal moan of forty-something women throughout America: Whhhy-y-y-y-y?

We Just Don't Move the Same Way

For starters, we're not as physically active as we were in our early twenties. Then, we were likely to go jogging, walking, cycling, and swimming with friends. Now, we're lucky if we get out of the car or move away from the computer because we're so focused on our careers and families, says Pamela Peeke, M.D., assistant clinical professor of medicine at the University of Maryland in Bethesda and author of *Fight Fat after Forty*.

"Many women are working and sitting on their bottoms all day long," says Dr. Peeke. "The lawyer becomes a judge, so she's no longer standing in court. And when she goes out, it's for a lunch meeting, not a night out on the town."

Then there's our kids. Lord knows we love them. But when you think about what they did to our bodies . . . Pregnancy often pads our bellies, hips, and thighs with fat that only daily exercise will budge. In fact, it brings one of our worst nightmares to life: It creates new fat cells that may *never* die. That's one reason why it often takes 10 years to lose the weight that we gained in 9 months.

And, of course, there's perimenopause, that 5- to 10-year period before menopause actually hits. During this time, our hormones are fluctuating as wildly as when we were teenagers. Only this time, instead of speeding things up, they're slowing things down.

Cheer up. There are many positive steps that we can take to slow down the normal aging process and meet our weight loss goals. They just require a little more of that wisdom and ingenuity that we've amassed with age.

Curling Iron

Muscle should be considered a hot commodity because it incinerates calories. Every pound of muscle on your body burns at least 35 calories a day; a pound of fat burns about 2. And that's just while

WOMAN TO WOMAN

Winning the Fat War

Ellen Kanz of Bloomsbury, New Jersey, first realized that she had a weight problem in the third grade. By the time she turned 13, she tipped the scales at 200 pounds. Disgusted with the way she looked, Ellen went on one starvation diet after another. Each time, the pounds came off, but she quickly regained them all—and then some. At her heaviest, Ellen weighed 225 pounds and wore a size 24. Today, at age 52, she is 50 pounds thinner and wears a size 14. She credits eating sensibly and daily physical activity with helping her stay fit and trim for the past 8 years. Here's how she did it.

I was 13 years old when I first started dieting. My mom took me to a doctor who prescribed prescription weight loss pills. From that point on, I started a pattern of losing and gaining 20 to 40 pounds by starving myself. That went on for years.

My weight problem was clearly the result of my eating too much candy, desserts, and fast foods. I love chocolate, ice cream, tacos, pizza, hamburgers, French fries, and onion rings. So every time I lost the weight, I'd start eating these foods again and gain it right back.

Finally, in 1991, I did something different: While living in Florida, I started eating sensibly and swimming about 100 laps a day. A year later, I had lost 40 pounds. It took a while to lose the weight, but I was able to maintain it. I discovered that if I make a commitment to weight loss and take my time, the pounds stay off. That realization never occurred to me before.

Now, I walk 3 miles a day five times a week. I limit my sweets and fast foods, and I focus on healthy eating. I eat bagels and yogurt for breakfast and vegetables, salads, sandwiches, and lean meats for lunch and dinner. I also drink a lot more water.

Despite my success, I'm still learning how to eat more healthfully each day. My goal is to lose another 10 to 15 pounds. And that's doable as long as I continue to walk in the right direction.

FAT CAN BE A GOOD THING

Did you know that carrying around a few extra pounds in your menopausal years can be an advantage?

If you're physically active, no more than 20 pounds overweight, and your additional padding is on your hips and thighs instead of your abdomen, you'll have more estrogen in your body than your thinner counterparts. Estrogen resides in fat, which may mean fewer hot flashes, less vaginal dryness, and a lower risk for developing osteoporosis, says Denise Bruner, M.D., president of the American Society of Bariatric Physicians and a physician practicing in Arlington, Virginia.

Body fat also offers some protection against osteoporosis by acting as a reserve bank when you don't meet your nutritional needs. "There are certain times when your muscles pull what they need from your fat stores instead of your bones to sustain themselves, which keeps your bones intact," says Dr. Bruner.

What's more, added fat preserves vitamin D, needed for calcium absorption.

"You literally go from being a metabolic furnace in your twenties to a glacier in your forties and fifties," says Dr. Peeke.

The good news is that we can regain every pound of muscle that we've ever lost, and then some, through weight training. Devoting just 20 minutes three days a week to strengthening our arms, shoulders, back, stomach, chest, and legs can help us build about one pound of muscle every month. After 2 months, our bodies will burn 70 calories more a day.

Add aerobic exercise like brisk walking, jogging, or cycling to your weight routine, and you'll burn up to an additional 300 calories per each 45-minute session. "It will keep you metabolically hot," says Dr. Peeke. "You want your muscles rocking and rolling."

you're lying on your back reading the latest *Cosmo.*

That's one reason why we could eat whatever we wanted when we were younger and still not gain weight, says Denise Bruner, M.D., president of the American Society of Bariatric Physicians and a physician practicing in Arlington, Virginia.

But beginning around age 20, thanks to a combination of aging and sedentary lifestyle, we start losing muscle—about 5 pounds every decade. By the time we hit our forties, we're burning 350 fewer calories a day than we did in our twenties. By our sixties, we'll be burning 700 fewer calories. This adds up to 10 more pounds of weight every decade if we don't change our eating and exercise habits.

The Hormonal Roller Coaster

At some point in our forties, that delicate balance of female hormones goes awry. Estrogen levels start to drop, along with progesterone, DHEA (dehydroepiandrosterone), and thyroid and growth hormones, all of which can dramatically slam the breaks on our metabolism. Here's how each affects our weight.

Estrogen. Falling estrogen levels can rearrange body fat. The fat that once graced your hips and thighs in your twenties and thirties suddenly makes a beeline for your stomach, changing your pear shape into an apple. Why? The less estrogen you have, the more you have of certain enzymes that make your stomach area suck up the fat.

Too much fat around tummies is toxic, says Dr. Peeke, because it can set us up for heart disease, diabetes, and cancer later in life. "So women have to be on the red alert to keep that fat down to a minimum."

Thyroid hormone. Your thyroid gland, a butterfly-shaped organ nestled at the base of your throat, is a metabolism regulator. When all goes well, the gland pumps out just the right amount of the hormone thyroxine to keep things running smoothly. If the pipeline slows, then your metabolism starts to crawl, says Eneida O. Roldan, M.D., chair of the American Board of Bariatric Medicine.

It's normal for your thyroid to produce less thyroxine as you age, says Dr. Roldan. "That's why it's very important for women in their forties to do some kind of weight training."

Progesterone. Produced in your ovaries during the second half of your menstrual cycle, progesterone actually boosts your body's ability to burn fat. It keeps your thyroid gland working properly and stabilizes blood sugar so that you're less likely to snack. Less progesterone, less fat burning.

DHEA. Shortly after you reach age 20, this anti-aging hormone also begins to diminish. By the time 40 rolls around, your body makes about half as much as it did. And that's a shame. The less DHEA you have, the slower your metabolism and the easier it is to put on weight, says Dr. Bruner.

What's more, DHEA stabilizes levels of insulin, the hormone that sweeps glucose out of your bloodstream and into your cells to be used as energy. Too little DHEA means too much insulin, which prevents your body from breaking

---

10 POUNDS LOST TO GAIN HEALTH BENEFITS

If your doctor says that you must lose weight, don't press the panic button. All you probably need to do is drop 10 pounds. That's all it takes to lower your blood pressure, cholesterol, and blood sugar levels, says Pamela Peeke, M.D., assistant clinical professor of medicine at the University of Maryland in Bethesda and author of *Fight Fat after Forty*.

What's more, the first 10 pounds lost will help you place less stress on your hips and knees and thus help prevent painful osteoarthritis. You'll gain more energy, boost your self-esteem, and decrease your risk of heart disease; cancers of the breast, ovaries, endometrium, and colon; and stroke.

---

down and using fat stores, and also increases your appetite.

Growth hormone. Like DHEA, growth hormone is abundant in our youth. It keeps our cells vigorous and active and maintains lean body mass, bone density, and a healthy muscle-to-fat ratio. But as we age and our supply plummets, so does our ability to burn calories without exercise. The muscle we lose literally gets replaced by fat, says Dr. Bruner.

With all these forces of nature working against us, it's tempting to just lie back and accept the inevitable. But just as you can control how much muscle you preserve—and gain—through weight training, you can get your hormones back in sync with various therapies that only your physician can prescribe, including hormone replacement therapy and synthetic thyroid or growth hormones.

Responsibility Overload

In addition to our jobs, we're wives, mothers, chauffeurs, housekeepers, cooks, and accoun-

SAY IT TO BE IT: TOP 10 AFFIRMATIONS

Just as an athlete needs to practice and train her muscles to be strong and in shape, successful weight managers need to practice and train to develop a positive attitude about their weight loss efforts. That's one reason many weight management programs use positive affirmations or "self-talk."

"In our society, there are many negative messages about weight, willpower, and body image," says Lisa Talamini, R.D., director of program development and nutrition at Jenny Craig in La Jolla, California. To counter these external negatives and retrain your mindset, practice saying or writing powerful, positive statements like these.

1. I can enjoy all my favorite foods in moderation.
2. I take the time to nourish my body.
3. Every time I eat a food, I enjoy its color, its taste, and its texture.
4. I can be more active today than I was yesterday.
5. Today, I keep my body and my mind in balance.
6. I reward myself for every positive change I make in my life.
7. I live by choice, not by chance.
8. I am learning to love my body and myself.
9. I accept myself just as I am.
10. I ride the wave of my temptations.

tants. Many of us also care for aging parents. That leaves very little time for ourselves. Going to an exercise class at the gym? Hah! About as likely as taking a spur-of-the-moment vacation to the Bahamas.

Playing these different roles adds up to big-time stress, another contributor to weight gain. Chronic stress causes our bodies to release the hormone cortisol, which sends fat straight to our stomachs, says Dr. Roldan.

Even women who are full-time homemakers are at risk, says Dr. Roldan. They're more likely to experience low self-esteem and depression, which can often lead to inactivity and overeating. "Some homemakers may be totally dependent on their families for their self-worth, and that changes once the kids go off to college." The solution is to put yourself at the top of your list of things to do, and don't feel guilty about it. Care for yourself the way you care for your family. Set aside time to exercise and unwind when you know you won't be disturbed. If that means getting up before your family rises, so be it, says Dr. Roldan.

"Let's say your mom is in the hospital with a broken hip," says Dr. Peeke. "Go visit her. Get her the flowers. Spend time with her. Then get out to the gym for 20 to 30 minutes or walk briskly around the hospital grounds. You'll recharge your batteries, and you'll feel better."

The Dietary Checkup

With all the stress and time pressures in your life, grabbing an extra piece of chocolate, a bowl of ice cream, or a bag of potato chips soon becomes the norm. And if dinner isn't cooked, you're more likely to drive to the nearest fast-food restaurant. Eating out? That's a reward for all of your hard work. After all, you reason, "I deserve it."

But those calories add up, and so do the pounds. "Fast food is convenient but very high in fat. You neglect to eat your fruits and vegetables, and so does your family," says Priscilla Clarkson, Ph.D., professor of exercise science at the University of Massachusetts in Amherst.

A food plan to help you cope with daily stress,

strengthen your immune system, maintain muscle mass, and produce a gradual weight loss looks like this:

Nix refined carbohydrates. This includes white flour, white rice, white pasta, white potatoes, white bread, and table sugar, which is found in cookies, cakes, and sweetened cereals. Their high-sugar content causes normal insulin levels to skyrocket, placing undue stress on your body. "Your insulin levels literally go up and down like a roller-coaster," says Dr. Peeke. "And if this happens consistently, you risk developing diabetes down the line because your body is constantly dealing with a boatload of sugar and isn't releasing a steady flow of insulin that you'd get by eating high-fiber foods."

Get the dark starches. Eat brown rice, whole wheat or spinach pasta, whole wheat bread, and sweet potatoes. Cook with monounsaturated fats such as olive oil and canola oil to strengthen your immune system, and choose low-fat protein such as poultry, fish, and lean red meat. "Proteins are the building blocks of muscle, so these foods will preserve lean mass and bolster your metabolism," says Dr. Peeke.

Time your carbs. Eat your high-fiber starches before 5:00 P.M. Even though they're chock-full of nutrients, they're also high in calories. "You'll never lose weight faster than if you eliminate the starches after 5:00 P.M. Your weight will peel right off," says Dr. Peeke. That's because high-fiber starches like rice don't come in single-serving packages, so we're more likely to overeat.

Drink the right liquids. Avoid alcohol. While there isn't any fat in alcohol, it's loaded with sugar and, thus, calories that get stored as fat, says Dr. Roldan. Gram for gram, alcohol provides more calories than carbohydrates or proteins: One gram of fat supplies 9 calories; alcohol has 7, and carbohydrates and protein each have 4. If that isn't bad enough, drinking even moderate amounts can increase your appetite and cause you to lose control over how much you're eating. So stick with one alcohol serving a day, says Dr. Roldan. Either a 12-ounce can of beer, $1\frac{1}{2}$ ounces of hard liquor, or 5 ounces of wine. The best beverage for weight loss? Good old-fashioned water. It's fat- and calorie-free.

A Little Help from Your Friends: Finding Support

In 1998 and 1999, more than 750 residents of Dyersville, Iowa, joined together to lose weight. In 10 weeks, without using starvation or fad diets, they lost altogether a whopping 7,500 pounds.

Their secret: They gave each other lots of support.

From the groups of 6 to 10 that met weekly to the thumbs-up signs they got each day from everyone else in town (population 5,000), the weight loss participants never felt they had to walk the path to their goals alone.

While it's doubtful that we're going to get an entire town cheering us on every time we drop a pound, we can—and must—create our own support network to help us meet our goals.

"Your ability to get social support is every bit as critical as understanding the foods you eat and their fat content and getting yourself more physically active," says Susan J. Bartlett, Ph.D., assistant professor of medicine at Johns Hopkins Medical Institutions in Baltimore and a psychologist specializing in weight management.

You Can't Go It Alone

Research consistently shows that a buddy can help you keep to a low-fat diet, stick to an exercise program, and lose more weight than you would on your own. You're even more likely to eat your fruits and vegetables if you get support from coworkers.

In a landmark study out of the University of California, Berkeley, comparing 44 women who regained weight they had lost with 30 women who maintained their lower weight, 70 percent of the maintainers sought help from friends, family members, or professionals when they had problems. Only 38 percent of the relapsers reached out. In fact, one-fourth of the relapsers had no social support at all.

"Social support is one of the best predictors of how you're going to do with your weight loss in the long term," says Dr. Bartlett. The reason, she says, is that to make these kinds of lifestyle changes, you need a cheerleading squad.

"If you're a mother, for example, you need a family who is willing to support you making these changes, willing to give you time to exercise, and willing to make modifications in their food and their eating," Dr. Bartlett says.

Support can be particularly important in maintaining physical activity, says Susan Kayman, R.D., Dr.Ph., project manager of weight management programs for Kaiser Permanente's northern California region. "Some women have the internal drive to run on their own and go to the gym and work out on their own, but the majority of us are not like that. Women are very social beings, and one way to get more physical activity into your life is to make plans to exercise with someone else." Then focus on socialization, not just the activity. That means walking with a friend, driving to the gym with a friend, or meeting friends at the gym. Without that kind of support, she says, we're likely to just quit.

Bobbi Schell, who not only helped organize the Dyersville program but also participated in it, still meets a group of friends every Saturday morning at 6:30 A.M. to work out. "I schedule my life to make sure that I don't miss it; it's so nurturing," she says.

Would she do it on her own? "Never," says the rehab services outreach supervisor at Mercy Medical Center, St. Mary's Unit, the hospital that sponsored the weight loss programs.

What Do We Need?

The type of support you need will determine the type of person you should get it from, says Kristine Kelsey, R.D., Ph.D., a research assistant

WOMEN ASK WHY

If the media says it's okay to be overweight, why should I bother losing?

No matter what you hear in the media, the number on the scale is still an indication of how healthy you are. Too much cholesterol and fat in your diet, and you run the risk of too much cholesterol in your arteries, which could block your bloodflow and eventually cause a heart attack or stroke. If you weigh too much, your body can't produce enough insulin to convert food to energy, and you may develop diabetes. And researchers don't completely understand why, but obese people are also at higher risk for cancer.

So when the media endorses obesity or being overweight, they're endorsing all the health risks that go with it.

Expert consulted
Jan McBarron, M.D.
Director of Georgia Bariatrics
Columbus, Georgia

professor of nutrition at the University of North Carolina in Chapel Hill. The four types:

Emotional support. You need someone to just be there and listen. This might be your best friend or partner.

Tangible support. You need someone to provide some assistance, like exercising with you, cooking with you, or going to the grocery store to help you shop differently. Look to friends, coworkers, or your partner.

Informational support. You need someone who shares articles and books they've read about weight loss, or who provides simple education, like the number of calories in a piece of pie. This might be a nutritionist, doctor, or friend.

Appraisal support. You need someone who

will tell you how great you're doing, encourage you, compliment you on your appearance. This may come from people you barely know in the office or neighborhood, or from friends and relatives who know of your efforts.

You may need all four, or just one. But whatever your needs, be sure to make them clear to the people you look to for support.

"That's the thing we're very, very poor at doing," says Dr. Bartlett. "We assume that everyone knows how to support us, but the truth is that what's helpful for me may not be helpful for you."

Ask yourself these questions: Do I need an exercise buddy? Someone to keep me away from the cookies and cake? Help avoiding the cake at office parties? Someone to watch the kids while I exercise? Someone to take over the grocery shopping so that I don't buy high-calorie snacks? Or someone to fix dinner so that I'm not constantly taste-testing?

Then be clear and specific about your needs, says Dr. Bartlett. "You could say to your husband, 'One way you could be helpful to me is on Friday nights, when I'm too tired to cook, decide in advance what restaurant we're going to so we don't just hit the closest KFC,'" she says.

What doesn't work is depending on someone who is supportive and helpful in the way *they* think you need, such as a friend who turns into the food police, constantly berating you: "Don't eat that, that's bad for you; that's too fattening." "Don't choose them unless that's the kind of help you want," says Dr. Bartlett.

THE TOP 10 THINGS PEOPLE DO TO SABOTAGE YOUR WEIGHT LOSS

10. Giving your body more attention. When the weight loss becomes noticeable, family and friends may compliment your new shape. If you're not comfortable with that extra attention, you may spiral back to old eating habits. Shift the attention from your body to your health.

9. Questioning your weight. Simply being asked how much you weigh, even if you've lost weight already, can be stressful. If you're uncomfortable giving out the number on the scale, tell your friends that good health is more important than focusing on weight.

8. Asking you to skip exercise. Your lifestyle change requires you to spend time being active, whether it's gardening or going to the gym, but that may mean spending less time with friends and family. If they're feeling left out, try to make active dates with them, such as walks or bike rides.

7. Ignoring your progress. Healthy weight loss comes slowly, and it can be frustrating when friends and family don't notice that your jeans aren't as snug or that you're not as tired when you climb the stairs. Remain positive by pointing out the small changes in your body and in the way you feel.

6. Giving guilt. Family or friends might be intimidated by your weight loss and could try to make you feel guilty about it by saying that you're losing too much weight. Assure them that you're the same person you've always been and treat them the same way you always have.

5. Negative feedback. It's hard to stay confident when friends and family tell you that you can't lose weight. While you can't control what they say, you can control how it affects you. "People have power over you only if you give it to

Choosing Your A-Team

What you're looking for are people who are going to cheerlead for you, help you through tough times, celebrate your successes, and understand your weaknesses.

them," says Howard J. Rankin, Ph.D., behavioral psychology advisor for the TOPS Club and author of *7 Steps to Wellness*.

4. Advice giving. They tell you how *they* lost weight, about the great grapefruit diet *they* were on, and how the only thing that got the pounds off *them* was a 2-hour spinning class 5 days a week. They mean well, but their continual advice is as annoying as your mother telling you how to decorate your house. Explain that everyone loses weight their own way, and that this program is what works for you.

3. Food policing. You reach for dessert after dinner only to encounter raised eyebrows. Such a judgmental attitude could encourage you to retaliate by eating even more. Remind your friends and family that you've made a lifestyle change, which is not the same thing as a strict diet, and which includes dessert once in a while.

2. Food pushing. This is when someone not only eats in front of you but insists that you have some as well. "Just a bite," they say. Prepare with a plan, says Joyce Hanna, coordinator of the Health and Fitness Assessment Program at Stanford University. Think through what you're going to say ahead of time, such as, "No thank you, I'm trying to eat healthier," and practice saying it in front of a mirror.

And the number one thing people do to sabotage your weight loss:

1. Snacking in front of you. Simply watching someone eat could trigger unplanned eating, says Stephanie Noll, Ph.D., clinical psychologist and director of the lifestyle maintenance program at Duke University Diet and Fitness Center in Durham, North Carolina. Staying focused on your weight loss goals may keep you from giving in. If you really can't take it, walk away. Consider asking your friends and family not to eat tempting foods in your presence.

"Do you have someone you can talk to when you have a problem? About things other than weight loss?" asks Dr. Kayman. "That may be the person you need."

Think twice before picking your husband as a support. Most of the maintainers in the University of California, Berkeley, study had to look outside the home, with more than half the women saying that their husbands were *not* supportive of their weight loss efforts. Some even sabotaged their wives' efforts.

The reasons why this happens vary, says Barbara Jacobson, Ph.D., a Seattle-based psychologist and author of *Weight, Sex, and Marriage*.

Sometimes a husband is insecure and fears that if his wife loses weight, she'll have an affair or leave him. Or he's overweight himself and becomes anxious about how his wife will view him when she is no longer overweight. Or he simply likes food, enjoys eating out, and fears the change that this weight loss program will mean for *his* life.

There's another reason not to choose your spouse or partner for special support in weight loss: "Men just don't get it," says Dr. Jacobson. "Their weight is not a complex issue for them. They don't have their identity all tied up in it. So it's very hard for them to give the kind of sympathy and support that women may need."

There is an exception to the husband rule: If your husband is trying to lose weight too, he could turn out to be a good ally. In one study comparing obese people who lost weight with or without their spouses, women who participated with their husbands did much better than women who participated alone.

So where do you find social support? Basically, anywhere you can get it, says Dr. Bartlett. "It could even be a relative who lives 6,000 miles away who e-mails you. You just need someone

TOP TOPS TIP

Her Husband Tried to Reward Her with Chocolate

When Tammy Hansen, 33, a science teacher in Rockford, Michigan, tried to lose weight, she discovered how difficult it was to get support from her husband.

She joined TOPS with a friend 7 years ago. They were both stay-at-home moms at the time and exercised or walked in the evenings. But when Tammy got home and faced her family, she found temptation everywhere, especially in her husband's "rewards" for losing weight: chocolate-covered raisins, her danger food.

"My husband is naturally thin and can eat whatever he wants without gaining weight," Tammy says. "He just doesn't understand how I struggle. So his idea of support is, 'Oh, honey, you're doing so great. Here's some chocolate.'"

At first, Tammy accepted and ate his gifts, only to feel guilty about it later. She realized that she had to make her husband understand how much she needed his help. She told him over and over again that she couldn't lose weight on her own, and that if there's chocolate in the house, she'll eat it.

It worked. With her husband's help, she lost 61 pounds and has kept it off for 7 years.

"Now he knows that when I tell him I don't want chocolate for Mother's Day, I mean it," she says.

being a support system for each other," says Dr. Bartlett. "It may start casually with one person mentioning that she wants to lose weight, and the other says that she does too, and they start walking together at lunch 1 or 2 days a week. Eventually, they're walking 5 days a week and doing other things together, like bowling or eating dinner out."

One Town's Experience

In Dyersville, the weight loss participants held weekly team meetings. They set up e-mail lists to encourage each other, came up with team slogans, and set team goals.

The team approach was critical to the program's success, Schell says. "There's safety in numbers. No one likes to think that they're the only one that has a problem." For instance, people who never exercised before began working out in the Dyersville recreation center. "This way, they could go with nine other people on their team and look just like everyone else," she says.

In a postprogram survey, one woman said that she wouldn't eat a piece of chocolate because she didn't want to let her team down. "But if I were doing it alone, I'd go ahead and eat it."

This group approach is one reason why weight loss programs like TOPS and Weight Watchers are often so successful, says Dr. Bartlett.

"When my patients come to see me, they get one view, one perspective, and one voice of encouragement. When they come to a group meeting, there are nine others sitting in that room going through the same thing that they're

who is reliable and who will be enthusiastic, encouraging, and positive for you."

That might even mean getting it from total strangers on the Internet. One study showed that dieters who received interactive guidance on the Internet, including weekly feedback via e-mail from a behavior modification expert and an online bulletin board to talk with others trying to reduce, lost more weight than those who didn't get any support.

And don't forget coworkers.

"I see all kinds of examples of people at work

going through. Someone who has gone through a slump and came out the other end is going to have much more credibility than I am."

To supercharge a group's effectiveness, build it with friends. In one study, researchers compared the weight loss success of those who joined a program with three friends with those who joined alone and were teamed with strangers. Ninety-five percent of the participants who joined with friends completed the 10-month program compared with 76 percent of those who joined alone. Members of the "friends" teams also lost more weight.

Once you've identified potential supporters, keep in mind that a support system is not a one-way street. You have to give to get. That means saying "thank you," communicating honestly, and expressing your appreciation, maybe even with a small gift.

"The best social support system is one in which I support you on something, and in return, you support me on something," says Dr. Bartlett. For instance, if your husband is supporting your weight loss efforts and helps you find time for exercise, then you support his fly-fishing hobby and help him find time to go fishing or take a fly-making class.

HOW CAN GROUP SUPPORT HELP YOU LOSE WEIGHT?

Comparing yourself with a supermodel won't do much for building your self-esteem. But comparing yourself with other women trying to lose or maintain weight will help you develop more appropriate expectations, one thing you need to succeed in your own weight loss efforts.

Sharing your weight loss goals with others in a group setting keeps you accountable and realistic, says Ruth Quillian, Ph.D., a psychologist at the Duke Center for Living in Durham, North Carolina. Because everyone is in the same situation, it is easier to find support and understanding in a safe and less critical environment. Here's how to make the most of group support.

Get help from experts. Try a program like Weight Watchers or TOPS. They have years of experience and thousands of success stories.

Lean on a leader. Negative thoughts and comments aren't necessarily banished once you walk into the room, but a leader can keep people's attitudes and comments positive.

Meet weekly. The more often you surround yourself with support, the easier it will be to reach your goal.

Look for a lifestyle program. The program you join should set realistic goals and focus on overall lifestyle, not just pounds. If the program recommends that you eat less than 1,200 calories a day, find another one.

Exchange numbers. Find a few women to network with outside of meetings and keep in touch daily.

Stay active. Moving around is important, so look for a support group that encourages exercise and even organizes group activity.

Set goals for indulgence. Schedule massages, manicures, and bubble baths, and encourage the other women in your group to do the same.

The Kind of Support You Don't Need

There's positive support and there's negative support—and sometimes it's hard to tell the difference. Like the husband who, when his wife lost 10 pounds, presented her with a box of chocolates.

It's called social sabotage. Dr. Kayman had

one client whose neighbor would always bring over pies and other baked goods. "Because this woman didn't want to hurt her neighbor's feelings, she would eat the pie rather than clearly saying, 'This is the worst thing for me right now.'"

"We wouldn't think of offering a drink to a recovering alcoholic or giving a cigarette to someone who is trying to quit smoking, but we actually act offended when we offer someone food and they turn us down because they're trying to lose weight," says Kristi Ferguson, Ph.D., associate professor of community and behavioral health at the University of Iowa College of Public Health in Iowa City.

That's when a woman needs to be assertive and clearly express her feelings and needs, says Dr. Kayman. "Women often have great difficulty in being able to say what we need because we're so used to meeting the needs of others. Many relapsers are women who didn't feel like they deserved to be able to tell the other person what they needed; they didn't want to hurt the other person's feelings." This isn't easy, and you may benefit from professional help to build up your assertiveness skills, she adds.

Remember, people can sabotage you only if you let them, says Karen Miller-Kovach, R.D., chief scientist at Weight Watchers International. "Sabotage is a two-way street. We all know food pushers, but I've never met one yet who literally shoves food down another person's throat. You have the right to say no and stick to it. A pleasant, but firm statement that you will not comply with the saboteur's request almost always works."

Sometimes the negativity is more obvious. Dr. Bartlett hears constantly from women whose families and friends react to their weight loss plan with a virtual roll of their eyes and the comment: "Again? Why bother? How many times have you done this now?"

And sometimes the negative "support" comes in the form of jealousy, says Howard J. Rankin, Ph.D., behavioral psychology advisor for the TOPS Club and author of *7 Steps to Wellness*, from people who say, "You're getting too thin," when you've lost only a couple of pounds.

Deal with these naysayers by understanding that everyone views life through their own lens, says Dr. Rankin. "You shouldn't be deflected from your goal because of other people's neuroses."

What Are You Doing for the Rest of Your Life: Maintaining the New You

You're so good. You've spurned short-term "diets" in favor of healthy living, learned portion control, incorporated exercise and physical activity into your daily life, and now recognize your emotional eating triggers. You've lost 20 pounds, feel and look terrific and, by all rights, should be resting on your laurels.

Well, don't even think about relaxing. Maintaining your weight loss may prove one of your greatest challenges. But that doesn't mean it can't be done.

From examining hundreds of women who have been successful not only at losing weight but at keeping it off, some weight loss experts have identified two key traits: a permanent behavior change centered on health, not appearance, and the old self-image changed to accurately reflect the new, slimmer reality.

Diets Fade, Health Is Forever

"If a woman has gone on a diet to get a boyfriend or to wear a size 6, she's likely to go back to her old habits once she loses the weight," says Fugen Neziroglu, Ph.D., senior clinical director of the Bio-Behavioral Institute in Great Neck, New York. If, however, her goal was to improve her overall health, with weight loss an almost unintended consequence, she's more likely to keep that weight off.

"One of the critical findings," says Anne Fletcher, R.D., of the 160 weight loss maintainers she interviewed for her book *Thin for Life*, "was that they stopped seeing what they did to lose the weight as separate from what they needed to do to keep it off. And in losing the weight for good, they took the focus off 'dieting' and put it on permanently adopting a healthy lifestyle."

There's much we can learn from their success.

Plan for problems. Even when a patient is doing well maintaining her weight, Cathy Nonas, R.D., director of the VanItallie Center for Nutrition and Weight Management in New York City, still works with her to anticipate problems.

Maybe the woman roams the kitchen after dinner. Today she's snagging "good" snacks like

WOMEN ASK WHY

Why shouldn't I weigh myself every day?

Your weight fluctuates daily, and the number on the scale may have nothing to do with how much you actually weigh, or with your fat loss or gain. The variables are the time of day you weigh yourself, the clothes you wear, and what you ate or drank the night before. Fluid retention can also make your weight seesaw by as much as 4 pounds in a single day.

Weekly weight changes are more significant, but you can still have variations that don't necessarily reflect a true picture. You may have a significant loss one week and then a half-pound gain the next week, but over the course of a month, things balance out. If you're sticking to a healthy weight loss program, monthly weighing should show an overall loss.

For women, of course, our menstrual cycles have an impact on fluid retention and weight. Often, we may have a regular weight loss pattern for a few weeks, then the week before or during menstruation, there'll be a change: a smaller loss, a plateau, or a slight gain. This is normal. And don't worry; the loss will continue when your period ends.

While you shouldn't weigh yourself every day, you shouldn't ignore the scale, either. Often, women go into psychological denial about their weight, choosing not to recognize that they've been overeating and gaining weight. What works best for most women is to weigh themselves weekly but focus on monthly progress.

Expert consulted
Laurie L. Friedman, Ph.D.
Deputy director
Johns Hopkins Weight Management Center
Baltimore

dinner? Once the woman can answer those questions, Nonas works with her to develop alternatives so that she can avoid this weak spot. So she might avoid the kitchen after dinner, change her usual habits by exercising in the evening, or eat a slightly later dinner. You can do the same thing. List potential weak spots where you're likely to fall into your old habits, like snacking when you watch TV or tasting when you're cooking, and then think of a solution to your problem.

Say okay to imperfection. One common element of weight maintenance that Fletcher found in her 160 weight loss "masters" was that they gave themselves permission to not be perfect. Who wants to go through life never again eating ice cream or chocolate or potato chips? "It's fine to eat those foods from time to time, and in moderation," she says.

So when you crave a chocolate bar, buy one, eat a little, and freeze the rest. We often desire just the taste of something, says Jeannette F. Jordan, R.D., prevention/detection education coordinator at the Medical University of South Carolina in Charleston. If you try to fill the craving with, say, a sandwich, or crackers, you'll still yearn for chocolate, she says. And you'll have consumed more calories than you might have with just the candy.

Get real: your real weight. Often, overweight people set fantasy goal weights that

rice cakes or carrots, but tomorrow it might be pie or ice cream. Questions that Nonas explores: Why is she in the kitchen at all? And why does she feel compelled to eat after are very difficult to maintain, says Fletcher. About one-third of her weight loss "masters" accepted themselves at a somewhat heavier weight than their original goal. "One woman, who is 5-feet-8-inches tall, got down to 140 pounds and felt like she was living in a cage, obsessing about every mouthful and exercising fanatically," she says. When the woman took a reality break and accepted a healthy (for her) weight in the 150s, she was much happier.

Be a journalist. If you tracked your foods to drop pounds, don't drop your pen and notebook when you've achieved your goal weight. "You need to periodically see where your calories are coming from to nip any problems in the bud," says Suzanne W. Dixon, R.D., a research epidemiologist and registered dietitian at the Henry Ford Health System in Detroit.

Stay in touch with the scale. Most of Fletcher's weight loss masters reported that regular self-weighing—at least once a week—was an important element in long-term success. "It keeps you accountable," she says.

Report in monthly. Each month, ask yourself: Have I been eating enough vegetables? Is my eating style something I can do for the rest of my life and not feel like it's a punishment? Is my activity level as high as it should be? Am I healthier?

Keep moving. In a study of weight main-

GUILT-FREE PLEASURE
Dancing the Night Away

Can the samba keep you slim? If plain or fancy footwork is part of your regular activity program, the happy answer is yes. Not only will a night on the dance floor give you a workout but it can also help your posture and your social life.

"If you're dancing socially all evening, you're getting a sustained, low-impact aerobic workout," says Jackie Rogers, director of dance and exercise for the National Dance Council of America. An hour of ballroom dancing is equivalent to a low-impact aerobics class.

The most rigorous dances? Polka, swing, and quickstep. In swing particularly, which has enjoyed a resurgence, you get "wonderful exercise," Rogers says. "You're away from your partner, moving more because you're kicking your legs and making motions that you don't do in the fox-trot or waltz."

Proper dance posture also helps keep you standing tall and hones your balance.

Socially, dancing is a great way to foster togetherness—or to find some. A night on the dance floor is a romantic activity for couples, Rogers says, but singles can share the fun, too. Dance studios often have group classes that students attend solo, finding partners from the class.

"Dancing as part of an exercise program is terrific," she says. "It's good for the body, good for the social life, and it's fun."

To start dancing, check local adult education programs, colleges, and commercial dance studios. Look for certified instructors with qualifications from a member organization of the National Dance Council of America (NDCA), the governing body for dance professionals in the United States. For additional information, contact the NDCA at (800) 291-8623.

tainers versus regainers, researchers found that those who maintained their loss reported lots of physical activity; more than half said that they worked up a sweat at least three times or more

TOP TOPS TIP

She Avoids "the Three Cs" to Maintain Her Weight Loss

When Roe Wiersgalla, 55, joined TOPS in 1997, she weighed 336 pounds. Now 146 pounds lighter and a 2-year weight loss maintainer, this office manager from Milwaukee found an absolutely foolproof way to triumph over temptation. When a "trouble food" beckons, here's how she responds.

"My downfall was what I call the Three Cs: cookies, candy, and cake. I absolutely love them. I love to make them, I enjoy serving them to people, and I managed to control my urge for them the first time I dropped a lot of weight, after TOPS. When I got to my present weight with TOPS, which is the recommended weight for my age, stature, and history, my doctor said that I shouldn't lose any more. I began to gradually eat more and more of the Three Cs. Psychologically, it was as though I had permission to indulge.

"Until March 23, 1998. I know the date from my food journal. That was the date when I ate 5,000 calories in sugar. Even while I was eating, I knew what I was doing, but I couldn't seem to stop. I panicked. A wave of horror went through me that if I kept up at that rate, in just a few months, I could put all that weight back on. So I resolved to make certain things completely taboo and not have even a taste.

"Now, I treat sugar like an alcoholic treats liquor. The big hurdle is the first decision: 'Am I having the sugar or not?' and I'm not. I won't even lick my fingers when I serve pastry to others. When I see plates of cookies at a party now, my response is automatic: I give them no consideration whatsoever. I feel absolutely in control of my irresistible temptation.

"I may have more of some other foods from time to time, but when it comes to those Three Cs, I just have zero. That really works for me."

per week. Just 30 percent of regainers reported that level of activity.

Reward yourself. Treat yourself for maintaining your weight. Whether it's catching a movie or buying a new CD, these personal incentives will remind you that you're doing great.

Match Mental Images

One key to lasting weight control is in our minds. If, when we were losing the weight, we needed to understand how we used food to deal with emotions like anger and frustration, then continuing this self-awareness is critical if we are to keep it off.

But we need to go one step further. Now that we've changed our bodies through weight loss, it's important to let our minds catch up to the new self. "Many women come to me after losing 30 to 40 pounds and putting it right back on, over and over," says Sally Ann Greer, Ph.D., a psychologist in Arlington, Virginia. The problem is that their self-images are stuck in the "fat" position. "When they lose the weight, there's a conflict between that inner image and the actual image in the mirror."

To make the two images match, we change our behaviors back again, says Dr. Greer. "We'll take the second helpings and not pay attention to portions. We decrease our exercise and gradually put the weight back on."

The remedy is a "tincture of time," says Jan McBarron, M.D., director of Georgia Bariatrics, a medical center for overweight people in Columbus, Georgia. "If you don't take a full 18 months to change your self-image, your weight comes right back."

Photos are a great way to flip the switch, says Dr. Neziroglu. At her clinic, patients compare before-and-after snapshots. Then Dr. Neziroglu probes for the traits or qualities ascribed to the different pictures. "When women look at the 'before' pictures, they may have such negative images that they call themselves disgusting," she says. Even when they see the "after" photos, some women still don't view themselves as thinner. "They might say, 'I still look fat' or 'I look better,' but rarely does someone declare, 'You know, I look good.'"

Here's how to help your inner image of yourself match your outer image.

Talk to yourself. While looking at your reflection in a mirror or while gazing at a photo of your slimmed-down self, utter positive statements like, "I like myself at this weight," "I am a good person regardless of my weight, but I prefer this weight for health reasons," "I feel confident that I am in control of my weight," and "I don't need to eat to cope with life."

Go easy on yourself. Because self-criticism and moral judgements about eating are so prevalent with overweight women, Dr. McBarron advises kindness—to yourself. "Do I still eat desserts occasionally, drink wine sometimes, and overeat? Sure I do," says the physician, who lost 70 pounds herself. "Do I beat myself up and feel guilty? No." Keeping weight off, she says, is a process, not a destination.

Update your inner image. Through the power of self-hypnosis—it induces a profoundly relaxed yet aware state—Dr. Greer urges patients to mentally see themselves at their new weight just as others physically see them. "Try to involve as many senses as you can in this imagery: How does it feel physically to be at this weight? How does it look? How does it feel emotionally?" The idea is to replace that erroneous but stubborn inner image with an accurate one. An audio tape such as *Edgar Cayce: Self-Hypnosis* will teach you the proper technique of self-hypnosis.

Dr. Greer also recommends consulting with a psychologist trained in self-hypnosis. To find someone in your area, send a business-size, self-addressed, stamped envelope to the American Society of Clinical Hypnosis, 33 West Grand Avenue, Suite 402, Chicago, Illinois, 60610, and ask them for a list of the psychologists in your zip code who are trained in teaching self-hypnosis to maintain weight loss.

Dress to thrill. Many women who have been overweight won't allow themselves a lot of jewelry, makeup or dressy clothes, even when they trim down, says Dr. Neziroglu, because they still have their old belief that these trappings won't make any difference. So she assigns her clients homework: Go shopping. She encourages them to buy new clothes in their new sizes and accessorize with jewelry, scarves, and shoes. "It changes the way they see themselves," she says. "For the first time in a long time, they feel attractive—and know they can feel this way regardless of their weight."

Techniques for Tough Times

A fight with your husband. A job promotion. Your teenager's failing grades. Next thing you know, you're standing in front of the refrigerator slathering mayonnaise on bologna slices and stuffing them into your mouth.

The stress of both positive and negative change can trigger relapses, says Susan M. Ice, M.D., medical director of the Renfrew Center of Philadelphia, which specializes in eating disorders and women's mental health issues. Women, Dr. Ice says, are particularly vulnerable to emotional stress.

Here's how to manage through these tough times without reverting to old, unhealthy habits.

Quiz yourself. Ask these basic questions: Am I hungry? Thirsty? Tired? Do I need a cookie—or a walk? Am I present for my meal, or am I allowing my emotions to distract me? Questions as simple as these can help you refocus on yourself, says Lisa Talamini, R.D., director of program development and nutrition at Jenny Craig in La Jolla, California.

Take time for you. Just as you block time on your calendar for appointments, schedule time for physical activity, grocery shopping, writing in your journal, or even just taking a bubble bath.

Surround yourself with support. Return to your weight maintenance support group, adviser, or buddy to share your fears, struggles, and issues. This is also the time to make sure that those close to you know that you need support, says Roxanne E. Moore, R.D., nutrition education coordinator at Towson University in Baltimore and spokeswoman for the American Dietetic Association. That way, your husband will know that you won't snap at him if he comments on your hand in the cookie jar. And his supportive words—"Honey, you seem to be going for cookies lately. What's really on your mind?"—could be just the release you need to close that jar.

Step back. If you find yourself slipping, say to yourself, "Okay, I'm engaging in old habits because . . ." and fill in the blank, says Dr.

REAL-LIFE SCENARIO
She Just Can't Help Sampling Delicious-Looking Food

Jamie, 39, is a gourmet cook. She would rather stand at the stove whipping up a great fettuccine Alfredo or soufflé than go for a night on the town at the swankiest restaurant. Her husband and kids adore her cooking. So do her friends. But being so close to delicious food all the time is a real challenge. She just can't help tasting her masterpieces while they're in the making. It always starts as a sampling of this or that. But before she knows it, she has eaten the equivalent of a small meal, and dinner hasn't even started! By the time she sits down to eat, she doesn't always have much of an appetite left, but she can't bear to see food go to waste, so she always cleans her plate. Her dress size, needless to say, has responded dramatically to her behavior. How can she get her sampling under control?

Like many cooks in this very common situation, Jamie isn't aware of how much she's eating, and that's one of the problems. One solution she could try is using ¼ teaspoon instead of a cooking spoon to taste things. That little spoon, which holds enough to taste for seasoning, won't pack in the calories like a loaded tablespoon.

Another technique is to use a separate spoon for every taste (which she should be doing anyway to avoid contaminating the food). As Jamie sees the spoons pile up, she'd realize how much she was really eating.

Neziroglu. "The answer might be "because my boss gave me a hard time, I'm feeling worthless, and I must have everyone's approval all the time." Challenging that erroneous thought—that we must be thought well of by everyone, always—will help us see a situation realistically and resume healthy eating.

Write it down. A personal journal that emphasizes feelings—not activities—helps women keep in touch with themselves, says

The kinds of food that she cooks might need some adjusting, too. If Jamie's delicious dishes are high in fat and calories, she might try lower-fat, lower-calorie items that are just as tasty. So many people are watching their weight and cholesterol levels that they'd appreciate these healthier meals, especially in social situations.

If there are certain foods that Jamie just can't resist, she can still make them—but with someone else around to help monitor her behavior. Of course, if Jamie is hungry when she cooks, the urge to eat will be stronger. So, if she's cooking for a dinner party at night, she should have a sensible breakfast and lunch that day.

Jamie's tendency to clean her plate is another factor. She should pre-plate her food from the stove so that she isn't tempted to go for extras. When the meal is over, she can freeze the leftovers immediately or use them the next day. If leftovers just go to waste, Jamie needs to correctly quantify recipes so that she's cooking for fewer people, not an army.

Expert consulted
Roxanne E. Moore, R.D.
Nutrition education coordinator
Towson University
Baltimore

Dr. Ice. That self-checking is critical to staying balanced when you're tempted to tip back into old habits. The personal journal can be part of the food journal discussed earlier in this chapter.

Relapse Remedies

Oops! That muffled thud is the sound of you falling off the healthy-eating wagon. It happens to the best of us, but it doesn't mean that you can't pick yourself up, brush off the dust, and climb back aboard.

"One of the key predictors of success in weight maintenance is how you handle a slip," says Howard J. Rankin, Ph.D., behavioral psychology advisor for the TOPS Club and author of *7 Steps to Wellness*. "You can either use it as an excuse to say that you can't stay on track, so why bother; or, you can recognize that it happens to everyone, and you can rebound positively from it."

Try to react positively, not punitively, if you've had a lapse, says Talamini. "The old, negative cycle would be to feel guilty, mentally beat yourself up, and drastically restrict your eating. What works, though, is tuning up your skills to take better care of yourself."

Here's how.

Work the numbers. If you fall off the maintenance bandwagon for one day or a couple, before you berate yourself, look at the calendar, says Dr. McBarron. "There are 30 days in a month. If you stuck with your healthy living habits for 25 days, you're way ahead of the game."

Develop fast reflexes. If pounds start reappearing, don't wait to respond. It's easier to lose 5 pounds than 10.

Set self-boundaries. Determine in advance your "manageable range" of weight fluctuation and have a plan to handle it. For example, at 5 extra pounds, you'll boost your broth intake to fill up before meals, or change the ratio of low-calorie foods to higher-calorie foods by adding more steamed vegetables and reducing the amount of meat. At 10 extra pounds, you'll go back to support group meetings or check in with your doctor or nutritionist.

Remember why you did this. "People often need to face a fearful situation before committing to making lifestyle changes. For example, seeing one of your parents die from a heart attack or being told that you have diabetes and may suffer other health problems if you do not lose weight is often all a woman needs to hear to start making positive behavior changes," says Moore. Write down your reasons and post them on the refrigerator door as a daily, in-your-face reminder of why you wanted to feel good.

Plan for problems. Since haphazard eating is a major cause of weight gain, go on relapse-alert status when your routine changes. An imminent holiday or trip is a signal to think about how you'll handle upcoming meals and temptations. To prevent any problems, Dr. Ice makes these suggestions.

- Structure meal times by eating at the same time every day.
- Plan other "nourishing" things to do at high-risk times, like taking a walk, reading, writing in your journal, talking to a friend, or playing a game.
- Don't eat meals alone.

Index

Underscored page references indicate boxed text. **Boldface** references indicate illustrations.

hunger and, 78
indulgences and, 89–90
lifestyle changes and, 11, 77
meal planning and, 81–83, 82
milk in, 85
planning, 154–55
protein in, 79
skipping meals and, 85, 115
vegetables in, 85
water intake and, 78, 83
whole grains in, 83
Dietary fat, 26, 79, 130
Dietary Supplement Health and Education Act
    (DSHEA), 148
Dieting
    all-you-can eat diet, 40–41
    Atkins Diet, 40
    banting and, 37
    bingeing and, 25–26
    body fat and, 38
    diet pills and, 148
    exercise and, 39
    fact vs. fiction, 39–42
    fad diets, 36–42, 37, 38–39, 40, 41
    grapefruit diet, 40
    Hawaiian diet, 38–39
    health and, 39
    Hollywood Diet, 40
    hormones and, 34
    lapses in, 47
    metabolism and, 25
    muscle and, 38
    myth about effectiveness of, 25–26, 26
    nutrients-are-bad diet, 41
    problem with, 37–39
    rapid-weight-loss diet, 41–42
    statistics on Americans and, 33–34
    water intake and, 78
    weight gain and, 38
    weight maintenance and, 42
    yo-yo, 25
Diet pills, 148
Digestion process, 114
Dining out
    American food and, 131
    calories and, 34, 131
    Chinese food and, 132
    desserts and, 135
    as excuse for not losing weight, 18

French food and, 133, 134–35
Indian food and, 135
Italian food and, 131–32
Japanese food and, 133–34
low-fat food and, 18
Mexican food and, 132–33
perception of, 129
portion size and, 129, 134
Thai food and, 134
tips for, 129–30, 130
wines and, 132
Dips, 117
Dresses, 62, 67–68
Drinks, 34, 81. *See also* Alcohol; Water
    intake
DSHEA, 148

E

Eating out. *See* Dining out
Eating schedules, 13, 79–81
E-C-A supplements, 144
Embroidery as weight loss tip, 110
Emotional eating, 71–76, 72–73, 74, 75, 76
    appetite and, 74
    changing, 75–76
    coping and, 71–72
    food journal and, 73, 111–12
    personal inventory of, 48–49
    personality types and, 76
    protecting self and, 72–73
    romance and, 74
    stress and, 46–47
    triggers of, 73–75
Energizer type of eater, 76
Energy, burning extra, 14
Energy density, 86–88, 87
Ephedra, 143–45
Essential oils, 16
Estrogen, 152–53
Excuses for not losing weight, 11–21
    children eat high-fat food, 18–19
    counting calories is too hard, 19–20
    diets don't work, 11–12
    dine out too much, 18
    family won't eat healthy food, 18
    gym is expensive, 13
    hate fruits and vegetables, 17
    health food is expensive, 17